Other Books by Dan Stark

Silence of the Bunnies Tales of Life, Love and Survival (2007)
Gelding Goliath An Insiders Account of the Destruction of AT&T (2012)
Vampires A Novel About the Legal Profession (2019)

Tewksbury Tales Press, LLC.
19 Wandering Oaks Way
Asheville, NC 28805

First Tewksbury edition 2020
Original published in the United States by arrangement with the author.

Book and cover designed by David Stark
Set in Adobe Garamond Pro by Lily Stark
Cover art by Shutterstock and www.123FreeVectors.com

ISBN No. 978-1-934160-05-3

More Muttering from the Rabbits

DAN STARK

Tewksbury Tales Press

TABLE OF CONTENTS

Dan Stark is a very funny survivor. The humor comes from his father, who was a very amusing designer and builder of nuclear missiles.

The fact that he is a survivor is the only conclusion one can come to by looking at his life. In 2009, he had a cardiac arrest while walking his dog. About 9 in 10 people die when their heart stops away from the hospital.

Then, in 2019, Dan fell and landed on his head! By the time he reached the Emergency Room, he could neither walk nor talk. Despite these and other ailments too numerous to name, Dan putters around in retirement, enjoying himself.

Perhaps he should have mentioned the only accomplishment of which he is genuinely proud: his two kids, Henry (37) and Lily (23), and his granddaughter Kate (4), the daughter of Henry and his wife, Rebecca.

In *Silence of the Bunnies*, I thanked my dear friend, Margaret Tuchman, whose "courage and grace battling Parkinson's disease has made me realize how light a burden illness can become when you spend your time, as she does, helping others rather than worrying about yourself."

This wonderful lady, this dear heart, died yesterday, December 16, 2018, making the world a slightly less wonderful place in which to live. Her death was caused by complications brought on by Parkinson's disease.

Margaret was diagnosed with Parkinson's disease in 1963. She founded the Parkinson's Alliance to raise money to fight the disease in 1999.

During the time I knew her, she lived in Princeton, NJ. At the beginning, her house resembled a busy train station, with all manner of people coming to talk to her. Towards the end, the number of visitors shrank considerably, as her increasing inability to communicate due to the disease's progression made her less accessible.

I believe I started visiting her in 2005, and was a regular until I moved from New Jersey in 2017. Though the frequency of my visits lessened thereafter, I continued to visit her every three to four months. This was not, as some have imagined, just visits to be a good friend. I genuinely enjoyed my time with her. She had a way of drawing me out, and giving me advice, that has not been equaled in my 67 years.

And, when her health made it too difficult for her to communicate, we each would be content to sit in one of the two recliners that she had side by side, and hold hands.

She was my dear, dear friend, and it saddens me that she didn't live long enough to see a cure for Parkinson's disease.

Disclaimer

Wouldn't it be great if these things really worked? All the people I might have inadvertently offended would have their cases thrown out of court! "Sorry sir, he does have a disclaimer on file, and yes, it does say he isn't liable for any offenses."

Until such time as such results do occur, let me try to limit the liability in the following way: I meant none of the bad things that might have been said about people, and even if I did, they deserved it! As for the people in North Carolina who might not like the reporting of their speech habits, allow me to say that I reported what I have heard coming from the mouths of people here, without endorsement of any kind.

My intent was to make people laugh and think. We need more of both.

INTRODUCTION

The following stories seem worth preserving. Yet, with my own health not the best, their preservation is in jeopardy. They are strewn about my office, sometimes on the hard drives of computers I no longer use. Once I am gone, my fear is that the stories, like a good wife in Egyptian times, will be buried with me. The best way to avoid that is to package them together as a book and publish it while I am still alive, which then becomes too substantial to disappear. That was the theory anyway.

All such theories went out the window on the 18th of October, the day of my fall. I apparently fell down the one stairwell that I had in my house. It was a staircase that I had planned to make optional within the house, (i.e., not part of a path to which I'd need access). It would offer access to two spare bedrooms, a wine-room, and a game-room. It also had double banisters. Finally, among the list of "almost" safety features, I had pre-built the framework of an elevator. It didn't protect anyone but it did make me feel virtuous for having thought ahead and planned for it.

In looking back at the fall site, I noticed that I had achieved pretty good elevation in the fall! I don't mean to complain, but this was from someone who could never get his feet over his head in diving class – here I had put quite a thump in the wall, and put quite a dent in my head. By the time they wheeled me into the emergency room, I could no longer walk or talk, and many of my bodily functions were beginning to shut down. Given my history with Parkinson's, embellished with my heart attack, spending much on me seemed to be a waste.

Things seemed be going badly across a wide array of activities. For instance I apparently had the sort of brain damage that caused hallucinations as I struggled to decide what was real and what was fake. In my case, the hallucinations were so real and so frightening that I lashed out at the hospital staff who found themselves holding on to me for dear life. It might not seem real now but when one is convinced that the staff are trying to tie you up in the car seats so that they can roast you in them, it seemed worth a punch or two to dissuade them from such follies.

In my view, such places develop codes of physical restraint well beyond the original justification. To me the original theories of preventing a person from doing harm to himself or others were redeployed as a widespread denial of due process, based on generalized observations. Lord help me if I were to place my feet on the right side of the bed! Each time I did I received the almost instantaneous response, "and where do you think you are going?" You'd think I had just insulted their gods, so hostile was the reaction.

The time with respect to the recovery and acceptance back into society was not something for the faint of heart. There were times when I felt such despair; thank god for the lighter hearted people who worked there who gave me respite from the doom and gloom I often felt.

PART I:

Parkinson's Disease

It is fair to say that my story, "Wired for Hope," left the subject of this disease with some optimism: at the time I wrote it, I had just undergone "Deep Brain Stimulation," in which electrodes were implanted in my brain, and I was experiencing a reduction in symptoms. Even though DBS didn't affect the progress of the underlying disease, it nonetheless gave precious additional time to the researchers to come up with something new, by postponing for slightly over a decade (in my case) the worst of the disease symptoms.

That precious time has now passed, and the underlying disease has come roaring back into view with a vengeance. I walk only with difficulty, when I do my trunk often is twisted. I frequently find myself going faster than I'd like or is safe. I'm not at the end of my bag of tricks either, but I feel less optimistic given the limited advances in treatment achieved over the last ten years.

Don't misunderstand me; I am not blaming or faulting in any way those doing the research. I accept that solving Parkinson's is a very difficult challenge that will take a very long time. It's just that my survival, irrelevant to most but of some importance to me, is being threatened by the current pace of progress, and the only outlet I have is to write about it. Which is what I did recently, for the Washington Post.[1]

---

1 The substance of "Ten Years After" appeared (under a different headline) in the Washington Post on September 29, 2017

First Interlude:

Ten Years After

I used to tell people considering deep brain stimulation — which involves the surgical implantation of electrodes into the brain — that it gave the typical Parkinson's sufferer perhaps 10 years of relief, during which the symptoms would be relatively minor. The bet — this is, after all, brain surgery that carries some risk of serious adverse results — would be that sometime during that decade, researchers would come up with a real solution. In other words, DBS was a way to buy time. Still, 10 years is no small period, particularly for those who have no other hope.

My experience is typical. I had DBS just under 12 years ago. Things went so well that I became a huge fan of the procedure.

But DBS works on only some Parkinson's symptoms. (Drooling, for example, is not affected.)

For slightly more than a decade, DBS performed wonders on me, eliminating the shakes that had accompanied my attempts to beat back Parkinson's symptoms with medicine alone. But because DBS masks the symptoms while not affecting the underlying disease, in the end it will fail the Parkinson's patient.

For me, the failure was in the form of a one-two punch. The first blow was self-inflicted. In April, one of the batteries powering my neural implants died. That was my fault; one should monitor the batteries and replace them in advance. Because I hadn't, I got a taste of what life would be like without the stimulators.

Swallowing became a problem. Taking my pills became an adventure. Some techniques enabled me to swallow a pill sometimes, while others did not. I became alarmed because I had had a cardiac arrest in 2009 and needed to take my heart pills. What if the swallowing problem became worse?

I wrote an email to my doctors explaining the crisis. Among the medicines I was taking were blood thinners that made surgery to replace the batteries highly risky. The doctors ordered me to go to the emergency room and wait until enough of the blood thinners had passed through my body to improve the odds.

I could barely eat, swallow or move, and I was in tremendous pain. The three days I waited were as close to hell as I ever want to get!

Fortunately, it was the stimulator unit on my right, which controlled my left side, that had gone out, which meant I still had some functionality on my right side. Being right-handed, I could still clean myself after using the bathroom.

As soon as the batteries were replaced, my body began to return to normal. The second punch was that "normal" started to change. It became hard to dispute that I was falling more — sometimes small spills that I could explain away; sometimes spectacular spills that I had to acknowledge. Taking out the recycling resulted in my losing my balance and ending up face down in the street. I was able to break my fall with my hands, at a price of fracturing my left wrist.

To limit the risks, I began to limit my activities. Someday I will write the definitive book about moving to a new home — a house in the North Carolina mountains — without lifting anything heavy for fear of losing my balance. Yet I managed, with the love and hard work of friends, like Pat Oakes, my daughter Lily, and my siblings David and Debra, who helped me move into my dream home — though, perhaps too late to fully enjoy it.

Postural instability is only one of the new realities. I also get stuck — I find it difficult to take a first step — fairly frequently. And when I do get going, I move my feet very quickly, galloping when I really wanted to move only a few feet. The first time I ran past my brother, I caught his unguarded expression, which said (loosely translated), "What more, dear Lord?" This is more of a concern than the drooling because, while both make me the life of the party, galloping also threatens my ability to walk.

I had my 10 years, and that was the deal, right? True, but that seems so hard to accept now. Despite all the wonderful work being done by the Michael J. Fox Foundation for Parkinson's Research and others — the government allocated about $168 million for Parkinson's studies in 2016, according to the Foundation — what has improved in the past decade? As one desperately in need of a different answer, it pains me to report that there is little more that can be done now. Oh, certain people get better results from the drugs they take, but by and large the treatments are unchanged.

At the risk of beating a dead horse, I am going to revive a proposal I made 10 years ago in my book, "Silence of the Bunnies." President Trump: Fund a $10 billion research effort to find cures for 10 diseases — a billion dollars a disease. Please make Parkinson's one of the 10. Attract the best minds possible, give them their mission of finding cures within two years, and then let them go without further red tape or prescription. Think of it as a Manhattan Project for

10 scourges that bring misery to millions. Imagine the good that could be done if a cure for even one of the ten is found!

It could yield a legacy that would last forever. And like all good deeds, it would create a swath of thankful people, too small perhaps by themselves to make a difference, but linked by family and friendship to many more.

For me and hundreds of thousands of people like me, it is the only chance we have left.

☆☆☆

Margaret Tuchman was a great friend of mine. When I first met her in 2005, it was due to the efforts of Carol Walton, her "Girl Friday," who had taken Margaret's request to find me – the author of "Silence of the Bunnies," and run me to ground. I was not used to being sought after, and gladly accepted the request to come to Princeton to meet with Margaret.

The first time I went to visit I remember the feeling of being in a busy train station. Margaret was a vital woman, busy with the day to day issues of running a small organization (The Parkinson Alliance) dedicated to finding a cure for Parkinson's disease. At the time we met, she had had symptoms for roughly twenty years, and I had only been diagnosed some years earlier. I went under the knife for DBS later the year we met.

I didn't go quietly however. My article, "Thoughts on My Upcoming DBS Surgery," appeared in Margaret's organization's newsletter.

Second Interlude:

Thoughts on my Upcoming DBS Surgery

In less than a month I am going to have my head put into some sort of Frankenstein device to hold it steady while a very smart doctor drills two holes in it, so that he, in consultation with a very smart Parkinson's specialist, can mess with my brain. I'm not really worried about whether they know what they're doing. They've done this to other people and those patients are alive, even improved. I worry instead about the neurosurgeon sneezing at the wrong moment. Sure you don't hear about it, but it must have happened.

I'm getting Deep Brain Stimulation, or DBS. I am not a medical expert and I don't offer any advice here. I'm going to be one more data point for those interested. I was diagnosed with Parkinson's disease almost seven years ago. While that is not a long time, I seem to be rushing through the early stages of the disease and sense I am heading for rough waters. I try to "Live Life Large," as I wrote in the Washington Post. I have too much I want to do during my life and I resent a disease that first limits, and then eliminates my opportunity to do it.

I have been labeled an "ideal" candidate for DBS. When I'm "on" I'm very on, meaning that when the medication is at peak effectiveness I can act very human. It just doesn't last long enough. Hopefully, the surgery will allow me to move my limbs without taking my daily dose of twenty or thirty Parkinson's related pills. Reducing the intake of pills should cure the involuntary shakes, rattles and rolls, side effects caused by too much medicine in the bloodstream.

Hitting a home run would mean being able to do simple things that most of you take for granted, like getting out of bed in less than five minutes, straightening my back before the medications I take kick in, or going to dinner without turning into a whirling dervish who nearly squirms out of his chair. Those simple things would make life so fantastic!

There is one feature of the operation that I don't like: you're awake during the entire time they're playing around in your head so that they can communicate with you. What fun. Just think -- six hours of having to answer the question, "Can you hear me now?"

Allowing your mouth to stay awake while your discretion and judgment have been put to sleep is troubling. There are some messy thoughts up there that I should have thrown out long ago. It is like inviting someone to your home, forgetting that you haven't cleaned it since 1965. Who knows what they're going to find?

My plan had been to talk about a safe topic like baseball. It's an old trick used by men when we start thinking about women that we shouldn't be thinking about. Force yourself to think about baseball instead. It never worked, at least for me. The law of averages says it's got to work sometimes. I had planned to at least give it a whirl here.

The problem is that my Parkinson's doctor is a Yankees fan and she knows that I'm a Red Sox fan. It's not that she would deliberately kill me, given that this is not play-off season. But she has threatened to change my allegiance surgically. I thought she was joking until, purely by accident, I found a manual on such a procedure locked with her private things in her desk. (I thought I had heard someone calling for help.) It's a diabolical book. Here's a short excerpt:

"Directions to convert Red Sox fans into Yankees fans:

Step One: *Remove and discard a minimum of half the cranial capacity of the patient. Patients with more than half a brain do not like the Yankees. After removal of the first piece, ask the patient a few simple questions. If he exhibits any critical judgment, remove more of his brain. Repeat as many times as necessary to produce a slobbering simpleton with the brain of a tapeworm, able only to mumble. "Did you see Bucky Dent hit that thing?" Then put a beanie on his head.*

Congratulations, you've produced your first Yankees fan."

Deep Brain Stimulation is a much milder procedure by comparison. There's really nothing to remove other than some bone and scalp. They then insert a few wires, which shoot impulses that, oh what the hell – I have no idea what they do. I don't really understand how this works. I am like the guy with the salami. I want to eat it because I like the result. I don't want to know how it was made.

I do wonder about one thing. I would like to meet the very first patient who had this done. What would make a person willing to have holes drilled in his/her head to try something that had never been tried before? Yes, it had been demonstrated to work and had been approved by the FDA. Lots of things work in theory. I took a long time making up my mind, even knowing this is a proven procedure and (I thought) that I had excellent and experienced doctors. Someone was willing to take a huge leap of faith that I admire but don't know if I could match. I stand in awe both of a disease that can stimulate that sort of bravery and the human being that stepped up to the challenge.

I am very lucky. I'm still in pretty good shape, meaning I can take care of myself. But I also spend a good part of each day out of commission. I do not absolutely require the surgery; I could limp along without it. So why do I choose to do it?

Surviving isn't enough for me. I am doing fine but I want to do better. My experience with Parkinson's instilled a zest for life. It made me realize how beautiful life can be. It did so by robbing me of the ability to do many of the things that make life so precious. Reminding one of the wondrous nature of life but then preventing you from enjoying it is one of the cruel ironies of the disease.

I intend to have the last laugh. If we can cure or at least hold the disease at bay, I get to keep the cake and eat it too. I get the wake up call to enjoy the wonders of life, and I also get the time to do it. DBS seems to give me the best chance to do that. Now that I've crossed the bridge and decided to have the surgery, wild horses couldn't keep me away.

My surgery is the first week of October. Given my gratuitous comments on the Yankees, I will not disclose the location. Look, I really don't hate the Yankees that much. There are games where they are playing a team in the National League where I don't actively root against them. I am even willing to risk emerging from surgery liking them, to get a handle on this Parkinson's thing. That's a lot for a Red Sox fan.

Wish me luck.

☆☆☆

Medtronic is the manufacturer of the DBS hardware. For a long time, they were the only company offering such a product. In my opinion, this had negative effects on the pace of their product development. In other words, with no competitor making them nervous, they weren't breaking their necks to improve their products. The batteries in particular, which had to be surgically replaced, had not seen an extension in operating life in the last decade. Imagine if they were in the consumer products market. I did, and came up with the following, again run in one of the publications of Margaret's organization.

THIRD INTERLUDE:

HOW TO MAKE A GOOD PRODUCT GREAT

It's hard to be helpful without people becoming suspicious. I hope the good people at Medtronic know that I am not being critical. I had Deep Brain Stimulation a few months ago, and have four pieces of your hardware in me: two electrodes in my brain, and two battery packs/controllers in my chest. That's not counting the wires that run under the skin between chest and brain. They are all doing fine, thanks.

That's not to say they are perfect, however. Consider the following suggestions as a down payment of the debt of gratitude I owe you for help restoring my life from the ravages of Parkinson's disease. I figure you are the same as everyone else – sometimes you keep your heads down and are just too darn busy working on the trees to see the forest. Here are some ideas that can make your products so attractive that even those who don't have Parkinson's will want them implanted!

1. License Rolex' Kinetic Energy Technology.

Your batteries wear out rather quickly. If I last more than three-four years, I am likely to require additional surgery to replace the old batteries with new ones. As one who has had his share of surgery, permit me to tell you that stinks! I have a better idea. Go to a good jewelry store and look at a Rolex watch. Guess what? It has no battery. If you wear it regularly, it will run forever. It generates the power it needs using kinetic energy from bodily movements.

This seems a perfect solution. The DBS electrodes are not electricity hogs. The average user of your product, even post-surgery, moves around a lot more than the average Rolex customer. One good bout of dyskinesia and we would charge the apparatus for months! If you feel your batteries are running low, you could just pop a few extra pills. By the time the shaking stopped, you'd be fully charged and ready to go.

2. License the Nano from Apple.

No offense, but your apparatus is really kind of big. I assume mine was correctly installed, but they still poke out of my chest, making me look a bit freaky. The size of these reminds one of one of consumer electronics -- a few decades ago. One of the great advances of modern engineering has been miniaturization. To catch up, simply license the iPod technology from Apple Computer. iPods are adding functionality all the time, yet they are both small and elegant. Imagine if the Medtronic products were no bigger than the Nano. It could easily be implanted into the chest without protruding in the least. You could have two of them as before, only now nobody could tell.

In fact, why not just license the Nano? It's programmable, and with a little ingenuity, likely could do everything your current device could do, only in a much smaller package. You could load your software, and then implant it rather than your current product. This will open other doors as well. Remember that the wiring goes from the chest, and wraps around the ear on its way to the brain. Perfect!

You could implant the iPod's smallish headphone cord at the same time as the wiring you now use, and just drop it off at the ear. That way, those of us with DBS would be able to listen to music on demand, right in our own heads!

3. Go Wireless.

I don't know who the industry leaders are in wireless technology, but you have only to look around to see that you don't really need wires to get from Point A to Point B. You could eliminate the need for wires altogether by working with someone with wireless expertise. It then becomes a smaller leap to allow the units to communicate not only with the electrodes in your brain, but with other people having the appropriate apparatus to send and receive signals from you.

Think "out of the head" and you may come up with something so nifty that even those without Parkinson's may want it. Once again, however, we are the lucky ones. Given that even your current unimproved product costs about one hundred thousand dollars to have one installed, we may – assuming insurance will not cover those who want it done for other than therapeutic reasons – be the only ones who can afford it.

You're welcome.

☆ ☆ ☆

As a result of some earlier articles of mine that had also appeared in the Washington Post, I was issued an invitation to attend a conference sponsored by the National Parkinson's Foundation, focusing on those who had experienced "early onset" of Parkinson's symptoms, which I believe they defined as anyone with PD symptoms who was 45 or younger. I would have qualified as an attendee on my own merits, being only 44 when I was diagnosed, but I couldn't begin to claim any honors for that, given that there were attendees who had first had symptoms as teenagers!

I had been invited down due to confusion as to who I was. The NPF had wanted publicity for the conference, and had hired a consultant to generate some sort of coverage for it. The consultant, innocently or otherwise, told the NPF (incorrectly) that I had a connection at the Washington Post and that if I wrote stuff about the conference, it was as good as in the paper! In any event, the consultant offered me expense money to come down and interview some of the attendees, and I, intrigued, accepted.

I did four interviews, and produced articles from three of those interviews. I don't know why I didn't write up the fourth session, but I didn't. I sent the three articles that I did write to the consultant, and only then did I realize that she had no intention of doing anything with them. I tried to get them in at the Post, unsuccessfully. Thus, the three pieces became orphans and – except for appearances in a few small magazines – they have not appeared anywhere. Until now. I am truly honored to be able to introduce them to the world, or at least the handful of miscreants who are reading this book.

One thing to remember is that the stories are based on circumstances in 2005, which is when the interviews with these people were conducted. I hope that all of them have been immune to the progressive nature of Parkinson's, but I haven't checked.

Fourth Interlude:

True Grit

If Cherie Zaun had been afraid of heights, she would have taught herself to fly and become a flight instructor. I do believe that she would have been the best damn pilot around, setting records for something meaningful to pilots.

I met her this week, not knowing what to expect. She lives near Hollywood, and is a very attractive, blonde professional golfer, still playing at tournament level four years after being diagnosed with Parkinson's disease. This disease attacks the link between brain and muscles, and normally affects those having it with crippling intensity. If sheer will could stave it off permanently, Cherie would be the one to prove it!

Yet Cherie is as likeable and enjoyable to be around as the girl next door. It is no doubt my East Coast snobbery that caused me to be surprised that someone who is all that she is still is so damn nice. The reason is simple – she excels at being human as she does at everything else, because she genuinely cares.

A colleague of hers reacted to my surprise by saying, "What did you expect? She comes from a good family and was raised right." There is some truth to that. She is a mixture of Tennessee and California rearing. She rode horses, professionally. Both her brother (Rick Dempsey) and her son (Greg Zaun) played baseball in the major leagues. Her father was a song and dance man who doubled for John Wayne. There is something in the bloodlines that suggested that this was the wrong person for the disease to try to push around.

In fact, since she was diagnosed she has fought back with grit and determination against an invisible enemy that caught her by surprise. To look at her, you wouldn't think she has Parkinson's. She has no easily visible symptoms, and still plays golf on a professional level with a bunch of "kids" who call her "Grandma." Yet from the day she learned she had Parkinson's, she has worked to turn her experience into something positive for others. For many, the long period of uncertainty and incorrect diagnoses before being told finally that they have Parkinson's is followed by an even more maddening period of what having the disease meant. Many doctors, and most lay people are not knowledgeable about the disease, and those that do know are often reticent about laying it out for the patient, fearing that the information will just depress them.

Enter Cherie. Since being diagnosed she has worked to share her experience and to make more information available to recently diagnosed patients. Cherie was put on a mild drug, generally used as an initial defense against the disease. (She is still on it, four years later, using a regimen of vigorous exercise and force of will to hold the disease seemingly in check.) Not at all content with the information available to patients, she wrote the company that produced the drug to point out what patients had to contend with to learn about the disease. I don't know what was said in the ensuing discussions between Cherie and the company. What I do know is that the company has since embarked on an educational effort and has produced materials designed to inform newly diagnosed patients of what they should expect. This is not a lady who crawls into a fetal position and complains to the universe about her bad luck.

The problem with trying to capture Cherie in a few pages is that she sounds too good to be true. A very experienced trial lawyer once told me that no matter how sophisticated a job he had done during trial, he would always turn his back to the jury and scratch his butt during his summation to let the jurors know that he was just like them. Cherie wasn't that crass, but the following morning, as she was leaving the hotel, she let her hair down and shared some of the possible advantages the disease might have. She made me laugh and realize that she was a down home girl who wasn't about to let a stupid little disease get her down or make her lose her sense of humor.

But I'll tell you a secret: she does understand that the best attitude in the world may not work forever. Every once in a while if you are sitting close, you can see her fight to control her emotions when talking about how her uncertain future may affect her family. To me, that made her more admirable than every other wonderful thing she has done. If she has fears about her own future, or wonders why of all people this disease picked on her she suppresses them, not because she is concerned that you or I might think less of her. Rather she acts without regard to such fears to show those of us in the midst of our own private fights against Parkinson's that it is still possible to live life joyously.

Thanks for the inspiration, Grandma.

☆ ☆ ☆

FIFTH INTERLUDE

TRUE LOVE

It is fitting to talk to Karl and Angela Robb together because it is impossible to imagine them apart. Those wishing to retain their cynicism about the continued existence of "true love" should stop reading immediately, because to listen to Angela's and Karl's giggling explanation of how they met and fell in love is to have all doubts swept away.

Let me start by being unkind. If Hollywood were making a movie about Karl and Angela, the two of them would be unlikely picks for the starring roles. Karl has Parkinson's disease, and his symptoms are not subtle. His speech is afflicted by a terrible stutter, and his balance is shot. He leans forward as he walks, making him look like a bull charging an invisible cape, even when walking a short distance. Angela is slightly heavier than the typical Hollywood heroine, and describes herself as being overweight at the time their love blossomed.

So what? In the looks exchanged between them, he was no less the romantic lead than Clark Gable; she left Vivien Leigh in the dust. It was their inner beauty that each saw in the other. "But surely," you say; "you might be mistaken. How can you be so certain that what you saw was 'love' rather than 'indigestion?'" Let me explain.

First, if they were merely putting on an act, they would have come up with a better story! Karl told people he had Parkinson's symptoms at age 17! Parkinson's symptoms at age 17! Who would believe that? His doctors certainly didn't – he was misdiagnosed for seven years before finally being diagnosed correctly. Then they claim to have met on an Internet chat room dedicated to football. C'mon! What was she doing on a football website? Her answer just piles improbabilities upon improbabilities. According to her, she stumbled upon the website while surfing the net in her office, on a weekend. What was she doing there? She had come in to polish her resume because her employer was moving to some idyllic location in Florida and she didn't want to go! In her words, she didn't want to move to some place with "sunshine and palm trees." Uh-huh.

Having met online, they next corresponded for several weeks before ever meeting. They disclosed between giggles that during the correspondence, the key "p" on his keyboard stuck, causing his messages to be filled with references to "pp," a fact they shared with me on the mistaken assumption that I would show some modicum of discretion and not repeat it. I share it with you now to convince any of you who still had doubts about the strength of their emotional attachment. It had to be exactly as they described it, because it is impossible, or at least inadvisable, to make stuff like this up!

Remember the blizzard of 1996, which dumped two or three feet of snow in the nation's capital? He had the flu, and when she learned of it, she took two trains, a bus, and then walked a number of blocks to come to his side. Then, when she opened his refrigerator and found it devoid of fluids she insisted that he must have, she bundled back up and went to a supermarket, more or less repeating her earlier trek before returning with flu-fighting juices and other things that would make him healthy again.

If I had received a call from anyone other than Angelina Jolie asking for me to do what Angela did for Karl, I would have done my best to speak in fake Chinese, adding in broken English, "long numba," slammed down the phone, and moved to Florida. Or at least I would have wanted to. The fact that she did what she did is evidence that their love for each other has no normal boundaries. A disease like Parkinson's that attacks the body is irrelevant if you are in love with the soul. He calls her his angel; she says he is hers as well. You'd better believe it.

Karl is nearly forty, and has had Parkinson's for more than twenty years. He has kept his humor and energy. He is a walking refutation of those who give up on love because of their symptoms. We limit ourselves for fear we will be limited by others, even when they are disinclined to do so. His remarkable level of energy has revealed itself in a series of business ventures. They also were co-chairs of the large and highly successful conference I was attending, whose purpose was to provide support to those who contract the disease at an early age. We laughed as we talked, and I left them feeling more invigorated and optimistic than I had in a long time. It could have been the Reiki demonstration he gave me, placing his hands on my shoulders in order to channel universal energy through his hands and into me. Or it could have been just being in their presence and enjoying people show a love for one another that makes life's little nuisances smaller still.

I recognize that this account talks far more about love than it does about Parkinson's. There is a good reason for that. Karl may have Parkinson's but Karl and Angela's lives are filled with love and only touched lightly by the disease. To write about them and focus on Parkinson's would not do them justice. They have used love, or universal energy to render the disease's role in their lives insignificant. Perhaps the rest of us, in between our traditional treatments, should take a page from their book.

☆☆☆

SIXTH INTERLUDE:

A MOTHER'S LOVE

I met Kelly at a conference hosted by the National Parkinson's Foundation for people who contracted Parkinson's disease while still quite young. In the week before we met, I met several ex-Marines, one a field doctor who at age sixty had to be arrested to get him to comply with the Marine rule against people his age being in combat, the other a veteran of several military campaigns.

If everything happens for a reason, I think I met those incredibly brave men to prepare me for meeting Kelly. She had fought an unknown enemy alone, starting at age twelve, without comrades and without complaint. Taking nothing away from the Marines, I can't imagine anyone braver.

Kelly didn't have much of a chance to experience life as a child. At age twelve, she was diagnosed with epilepsy. She battled it for six years and, miraculously, beat it. At age eighteen, she tested free of that disease. A year later, then nineteen, she became a factory worker, making auto parts. A number of solvents, some of them quite toxic, are used in the manufacturing process. At age thirty, Kelly started dragging her left leg when she walked. She sought medical help, and was told it was nothing serious. Later, she was told that she had Multiple Sclerosis. It took another year from the MS diagnosis for the correct diagnosis to be made -- she had Parkinson's disease.

Mistakes of diagnosis are disturbingly commonplace among those who start experiencing symptoms at ages younger than the doctors think that the disease should strike. Seldom, however, does the initial diagnosis have the ironically wonderful effect that it had on Kelly and her husband. They greeted the news that there was nothing seriously wrong by deciding to start a family. Nikki, her daughter who Kelly describes as the "Light of my life," was born a year later.

To hear her words melt with emotion when she talks about her daughter, and then to hear her say that she might not have had a child had she known she had Parkinson's, is to begin to understand the horrible toll this disease takes on families. There is not an ounce of selfish thought in her statement; there is only heartrending concern for the impact her disease will have on her daughter's life. Now, she says, it limits the energy and creativity she has to play with her four year old. But her real fears are for the future, when the disease's progression will reduce her abilities further. It is when she talks about this that cracks in her composure appear. Sitting in her presence as she talked revealed a glimpse of the raw power of maternal love. The fears for the future, so intensely visible for a moment, are transformed into a lioness' determination, etched in the set of muscles around her jaw, to fight the disease and not let anything harm Nikki.

Learning what lies ahead should not be so difficult! Allow me to complain on her behalf, since she will not, that it is unfair for her to have to plan a future without being given all the knowledge that the medical community has about what lies ahead.

Never being permitted to be a child, she has earned the right to be treated like an adult. All is not bleak. No, we don't have a cure, and the ability of current treatments to keep Kelly, now thirty-seven, functional for the rest of her life is imperfect. But she is only on Mirapex now. There are years of life in current therapies, drugs like Sinemet, and procedures like Deep Brain Stimulation. In the hands of good doctors, these tools will see her through Nikki's growing into a woman. Beyond that is the hope for better therapies, and the ultimate hope for a cure.

The lesson I derive from talking to this wonderful woman is not which pills she took or when she took them. She stands for much more than that. She is a beacon of inspiration that her love for her daughter can put in perspective the problems of parenting as a Parkinson's patient. No, she can't do everything for her daughter that those without the disease can. So what? How many parents do everything for their children that they could? Having met Kelly, I cannot believe that her daughter will receive anything less than one hundred percent of what she can do. And that is huge!

Sometimes our children are born with medical issues. Do we love them any less? If you show them love, do you think they might love you less because of medical issues you might have?

Nikki is one lucky little girl.

☆☆☆

Margaret Tuchman and I were good friends from the day we met. I mentioned earlier that her home had the feel of a busy train station. Over the years, I watched helplessly as the disease limited her ability to communicate. The hustle and bustle of only a few years ago turned into a sense of isolation, despite her mind being as sharp as ever.

One of my concerns about moving from New Jersey was that I didn't want to lose touch with Margaret, both for her sake and mine. I made several visits to see her. The visits were not raucous events; they were quiet affairs where I stayed for a few hours sitting next to her, while I told her what was going on with my life. I am not free of the progressive nature of the disease, and I leaned on my daughter to drive me to Princeton.

This next interlude was based on an e-mail that I sent her following my visit.

Seventh Interlude

A Letter to Margaret

At the end of my last visit, you leaned over and asked in a typical Margaret whisper that I "write you." I hadn't forgotten; I was just waiting to see if anything worth reporting would happen. Nothing of moment comes to mind. Just life. So I then had either to not write, or else to lower my standards of what I would write about. As usual, I chose to lower my standards, putting together the type of trivia that isn't worth mentioning into a sort of "day in the life mosaic."

Monday morning started a bit rough. The power went off at slightly before five in the morning, a fact that the power company insisted on bringing to your attention — repeatedly — text after text. They obviously wanted to share your pain, and went above and beyond what is necessary, keeping your smart phone humming, chirping or playing whatever tone you foolishly selected long ago to signify the arrival of text messages.

Normally, the power is knocked out by a storm toppling trees on vulnerable power lines, something for which you can normally prepare if you keep in touch with weather forecasts. For instance, I know enough to put flashlights within reach when storms are in the area. This time, the weather was fine, the cause was "equipment failure," and the surprise was complete.

I sleep in a recliner, with the electric powered chair tipped back nearly all the way. Normally, the first thing I do each morning is to restore the setting to a sitting position, from which I then — with some difficulty — climb out. Without power, this became a real battle. Eventually, I managed to climb out. There was still a good hour to sunrise, meaning my world was totally dark until then. Being in a relatively new house, I didn't yet know my way around absent some amount of light. I wasted precious time looking for my flashlights (which had been moved to an equally logical but different spot by my cleaning person the previous week). I had no choice but to try to find my way to the bathroom in total darkness, proceeding very slowly to avoid tripping on something, or falling. I nearly made it, and consoled myself with the thought that at least I had made it past the oriental rug to the tile floor of the bathroom before wetting my pants.

Tuesday, the highlight of the day is going to boxing physical therapy. It helps a lot, at least I think it does, but leaves me exhausted. My brother surprised me at the end of his day by stopping by and suggesting we go get sushi for dinner. Asheville rarely disappoints, and tonight was no exception. The sushi was wonderful. A new high point!

Wednesday. Went to physical therapy today, and caused havoc. I had a ten o'clock appointment but I thought it was at nine o'clock. I went there at nine, and went straight back to the exercise area as is my habit, and began warming up on the exercise bike. My therapist, Ellen, was suckered in by me, and worked with me, until her real nine o'clock patient ruined everything by asking where her therapist was anyway. They were still trying to sort things out when I smiled nicely at everyone, and left.

Which brings me current, except for the nearly two hours I've spent trying to type this piece up. I made the mistake of starting to type it on my Apple laptop, which is a hellish contraption better suited to being a table weight than a typewriter. The problem is that the keypad is located where the chance of me inadvertently brushing against it while typing is very high. When one does brush against it, a number of things may happen – all of them bad. It may choose to move where you are typing, or it may highlight previously typed text so that the next key typed replaces the highlighted text! My own view, after extended experience with it, is that it has a nasty little mind of its own, aimed to thwart honest reporting of how bad a word processor it is!

Love, Dan

☆ ☆ ☆

PART II:

AN AUTOBIOGRAPHICAL INTERLUDE

It occurred to me that I have been so busy getting dragged in different directions by the various interludes that I was in danger of leaving a gaping hole in what was an interesting but incomplete health history. To put this in perspective, remember that I was diagnosed with Parkinson's disease in 1997, had open heart surgery in 2000 to fix a leaky valve, followed by brain surgery in 2005 to deal with the increased symptoms of Parkinson's through placing electrodes in my brain.

But that leaves out two little incidents: first is the heart attack on July 4, 2009; and second is the Fall, on October 18, 2019. I shouldn't have survived either, and yet, I survived both.

EIGHTH INTERLUDE:

THE AMAZING CIRCUMSTANCES SURROUNDING MY CARDIAC ARREST

On July 4, 2009, I was taking a walk with my dog Coop when my heart stopped. I had no warning — I felt fine. My memory was snuffed out the same moment as my consciousness, and what I write about it now has been reconstructed with the help of others. I had an obstruction so that blood was not getting through to my heart. I fell to the ground; Coop sat by my side. At that point, my life wasn't worth a plugged nickel; even if someone had seen me fall and had immediately called 911, I would have been dead by the time the rescue squad arrived. And, even if one survives, the damage done to the brain and organs from those precious minutes without oxygen leaves you a vegetable. According to data kept by the American Heart Association, roughly 9 out of 10 people who suffer a cardiac arrest outside of a hospital do not survive; and the tenth person who does make it is rarely unscarred.

My angel's name was Mary. I know this only because she stopped me on one of my walks with Coop months later and told me what had happened. As she was driving to work on July 4th, she saw me fall. She got out and immediately gave me CPR. Someone else saw her stop, came to investigate, and called 911. The crew that responded to the call included Mark Rosenblum, a former colleague of mine from the AT&T law department who knew all about my health history and was able to inform those who needed to know what they were dealing with.

The first half hour, which is so critical when one has a heart attack, was near magical in my case. You could not script more timely or better care. By the end of that half hour, I arrived at Morristown Memorial, a hospital that has made heart care a core competency. Someone made the decision to put me into an induced coma, reducing my body temperature in order to protect my organs from damage during the recovery phase. Whatever they did worked and the first thing I remember of the entire episode was waking up in the hospital, to be greeted by friends, neighbors and family.

I have always been in control of my faculties and incorrectly assumed that I was still. At least I don't remember being warned that one of the side effects of coming out of a coma was that things were not always as they seemed. I was totally convinced that I was not a victim of a heart attack, but rather a near victim of a plot by a beautiful and murderous blonde who had married me over the weekend and was now trying to kill me in order to raise funds for her nearly defunct horse farm! So detailed were my descriptions of the events, and so insistent was I that this in fact had happened that my son, who I had placed in charge of my affairs as the most level headed relation I had, went online to check out marriage licenses. Nada.

A second hallucination rounded out my post-coma behavior. I was once again totally taken in, this time by the "I was a finalist in a game show" delusion. My last challenge was to persuade my son to go into the stairwell outside my hospital room, and sing, while holding an empty gallon water jug over his head. He complied, to humor me, and to his credit has kept his reminders to me of these episodes to an absolute minimum. Of course, he could just be hedging his bets in case I suddenly win the grand prize in the game show.

It was only a couple of days from regaining consciousness to agitating to get out of the hospital. Yes, they saved my life. But I am convinced that, given enough time, they would find a way to take it back.

When I think back on the heart attack, I can't explain with logic why it is that I am still alive. There are so many things that could have turned this day into my last. What if Coop hadn't chosen that exact minute to want to go for a walk? I live alone, and a cardiac arrest inside my home would have been fatal. Same result if Mary, my savior nurse, had left a minute sooner or later for work that morning. My continued existence is highly improbable. And, to be cherished!

How did I celebrate my survival? I went to my beloved Virgin Islands, where the weather is boringly beautiful, the bikinis breathlessly small, and my imagination just as robust as ever. There is something about the air and water there that washes my writer's block away. This time I hadn't thought it would work – the disruption in my writing had been too long, too severe. I therefore gave myself a week to write what became "Ten Years After." I wrote it the first night. Now that is cause for optimism!

I wrote those words the week before Hurricane Irma turned the Virgin Islands into a war zone. It is difficult to understand God's wrath sometimes. The place is without evil intentions; it is just a place of incredible beauty, the only drawback being that many who live there do so in poverty. I become angry as I look at the pictures of devastation, until I remember there's no one to get angry at. Then I just get sad.

☆☆☆

NINTH INTERLUDE:

THE FALL

I fell on an interior stairway, and did so with enough velocity to seriously mess up my brain. The only thing I can think of is that I must have gone looking for a bottle of wine to have before Jen and I walked up to my brother David's house for his birthday dinner. There was a serious discussion about whether to revive me, although to be fair I wasn't a good candidate because North Carolina has strict laws that I didn't satisfy because my heart was beating.

Other than that, not much was operational: I couldn't walk, talk, make noise or frankly communicate in any way. I had suffered a subarachnoid hemorrhage. I was a lump. I ended up in a rehabilitation clinic where a team started training me on basic skills, such as movement skills, speaking skills, cognitive skills. At the beginning, my skills were totally rudimentary. But factor in a desire for life, and I soon began an amazing record of progress, speaking in hackneyed

English, making improvements in a whole variety of physical talents. I worked tirelessly at it, and threw in chess to make certain that my cognitive function did not lag. (My chess playing was fine as Tristan would complain – I didn't lose a single game of the nine we played).

With respect to exiting from my fall, it's not so easy as learning to walk. When I wrote this, I still haven't made it home. It's a question of patiently following the rules, something I've never been very good at. At the end of the day, though, the rules will work, spitting you out and returning you to your home. I know this to be true – since I have been home now for nearly a week!

It doesn't hurt to have a skilled person watching over you, to make certain the rules are followed. In my case, my ex-wife Mary did such an excellent job, using data to keep the staff of the center on base! My survival is testament to how good a job was done here. I don't want to pretend that this was all or even nearly all of this was achieved as a result of external watchers. I had a great internal team as well. With apologies for any errors I may make in the list, among my favorites are:

Shawntale Harper: a true original! She had proposed we go on an RV adventure when I finished this, taking her son, to Dallas, where my son, daughter-in-law, and granddaughter lived, then winging west to Santa Barbara where my best friend John lived.

Jenn: the most amazing speech pathologist, who learned to love the Mills Brothers from me during a therapy session.

Melissa: a real protector of mine who helped me find my way through the sometimes ugly stuff below the surface.

Melisa: a sweet woman, who had the misfortune of standing in front of me when I, in a tribute to my mental state of health, pulled my PEG tube out.

Kelly: a wonderful occupational therapist, who gave me courage to keep going by telling me at a low point that I was special.

Alex: an uncommon expert who combined expertise at her craft with a real human touch.

Tristan: lest he go down as a chess player only, he was also a student of life's tangles who knew wisdom when he saw it.

Courtney: someone who was there from day one, who was dedicated to my care.

(This next part was written shortly before my return home.)

I will celebrate as soon as I get home. As of now, that depends on the views of two coaches that are appraising my work,

Steve and Hillarie: my coaches at the Lodge at Mills River, the last place I stayed before returning to my home. They confused me with someone with the energy to engage in crazy antics, which were dangerous of course, much to the fears of my family. All joking aside, they were wonderful!

The speed at which my recovery took place was noted on many occasions. The hard work, the refusal to accept the limited view of my capabilities shared by many staff, and even family and friends, was a product of the desperate desire to escape! I certainly was unaware of the great peril I was in, with the invasion of the country by viruses making life much more difficult, especially in places such as the rehabilitation centers where I was staying. But when one realizes that I was released in mid-February of 2020, after the invasion had started, but about a month before we became aware of it, it is possible to appreciate that any lesser speed would have landed me right in the middle of the Covid 19 mess! Thank you, Lord, for this not-so small favor!

☆☆☆

Tenth Interlude:

One Thing Leads to Another...

There were other events affecting my health in addition to the life threatening events described above. One such event began innocently enough, at the YMCA, where I was pedaling on the stationary bike. I had lost track of time, though it was something north of thirty minutes. Suddenly, my built in defibrillator went off, knocking me off the bike. I had assumed that the device would only be triggered if my heart failed. This was a not-so gentle correction of reality; it would go off depending on how it was programmed, and I had obviously crossed the line as to what had been assumed about my heart rate.

Did I say that the device went off once? No, it went off seven times! Each time it knockd me off my feet. Who knows how many times it would have continued to discharge its electronic spanking. What I remember was that a doctor who had an office in the same building as the YMCA, and had stopped to see what was going on. He told the YMCA staff to give me oxygen. It worked.

I was convinced of the need to determine why this had happened. Everyone had their theories. My cardiologist told me I needed to have a procedure to figure out whether I had a blockage. He told me that he no longer did such things himself, but that he had a colleague who he would strongly recommend. I decided to proceed. To his credit, the colleague came and told me that he had made a mistake during the procedure, nicking an artery in my groin.

For the next few days, I was told that I should move as little as possible, lying flat on my back in bed. I did so, and this played a role in causing my next crisis: my prostate somehow perfected its grip on my urethra, translating the inactivity to a limited ability for my body to pee. This in turn caused me to visit the ER, to deal with the pain caused by my swollen bladder.

The problem is that the only way to determine whether one can pee is to try. That means taking the catheter out, which means that the bladder becomes painful (assuming you can't pee) until you can once again insert a catheter. Inserting a catheter is clear hell! It is an unmitigated piercing shot of pain, followed by a surreal feeling of peace as the urine drains and the bladder ceases becoming the center of all pain in your universe. I spent the next year cycling between catheters and failed efforts to pee. Finally, my doctor advised me that I was out of non-operative options. He recommended that I consider surgery to pare down the offending prostate.

Fortunately, his proposal was blocked by my cardiologist, ostensibly because he didn't want me to have surgery just then. It did give me time to get a second opinion. Enter Sidney Goldfarb, a man who I will identify by name because he was the hero of my story here. Simply put, he looked at my prescriptions, changed them all, and within two weeks I could pee!

How is that for a happy ending?

☆☆☆

PART III:

TALES OF BEGETTING

There is nothing so cleansing of spirits than a total change of pace.

ELEVENTH INTERLUDE:

FROM THE BELLY OF THE BEAST

Dr. Dog was a veterinarian by trade. Of course, that's not his real name, but on advice of counsel, I have elected to protect his identity. He had an uncommonly successful practice, owing it to his hunkish good looks. He was dark complected, fit and had a full head of hair – not bad for a man in his early forties.

His clientele was a testament to his charms. A visit to his waiting room made it obvious that something was afoot. It was crowded at waist level, but it was standing room only at hip and bust level. The women would come, dressed to kill, bringing their sick or not-so-sick pets with them. Their clothing, gossamer garments that did more to reveal rather than conceal their beauty, advertised their availability in very unsubtle ways.

The doctor succumbed fairly frequently. He was human; he cannot really be blamed. With a pinch here, a caress there, he tried to keep his customers satisfied.

He pursued his amorous adventures with the tacit understanding of his wife. Their love had worn out, and she stayed with him because she had grown accustomed to the level of comfort the marriage provided. So long as he didn't make it so obvious that she couldn't pretend that she didn't know, their unromantic arrangement worked.

It was their dog, that we'll call, "Fluffy," that upset this delicate balance.

Fluffy had not been himself, a fact noticed immediately by Mrs. Dog upon her return from her yoga retreat. In fact, he could barely rise and his stomach looked swollen. Cursing her husband for not being more observant, she tucked her Armani pajamas top into her Armani pajamas bottoms, threw a robe over both, and ran out the door, dog in hand. Well, she actually made a small detour in this otherwise headlong race to save Fluffy. As Mrs. Dog was moving at a very commendable pace towards the front door, her eye happened to catch her reflection in the large mirror they kept in the foyer. She stopped in her tracks, muttered something about showing the bitches a thing or two, and put the dog down gently on a chair. Then she fixed herself up, putting on bright red lipstick, kissing the air in front of her as she pushed her bottom out behind her. "Grrrr," she said, liking what she saw. She ran a brush through her hair ever so quickly, grabbed the dog, and resumed her life or death mission.

Her husband was surprised to see his wife in his office, a place that they both recognized to be part of his domain. But when X-rays indicated the dog had a blockage, he overlooked the transgression, saying in a serious but caring voice, "Honey, the dog has a blockage. I have got to operate immediately." Then he turned to his assistant, saying, "Right, let's get going. Cancel my other appointments. We operate in ten minutes!"

His take-charge manner comforted Fluffy, while having almost a toxically aphrodisiac effect on some of his clients. A brunette with an impossibly small waist to go with her other body parts, was heard to tell her neighbor, "I just love it when a man takes charge, don't you?" Sadly, the reply was not overheard, because the woman uttering it had had a Hollywood career, appearing in several beer commercials, and was recognized as being a profound thinker who said important things.

"The operation was a success!" Dr. Dog's assistant announced a short while later to a still packed waiting room. "Mrs. Dog, you may go back now and see Fluffy. As for the rest of you, you are welcome to stay, but the doctor won't resume seeing other patients for at least a half hour." With that, she led Mrs. Dog back to see Fluffy. Not a single client took the news as reason to leave. What was time, if they couldn't use it to tell the doctor how much they admired him?

The doc's good deed, for his skill had saved Fluffy's life, did not go unpunished. In response to what had been the cause of the dog's distress, Dr. Dog held up a woman's thong. (By "thong" we mean that skimpiest of undergarments, not the rubber beach shoes.) "He had eaten this," the doctor said." The doctor said. "You should be more careful about leaving your things around, particularly after you've worn them and they are covered with your scent."

Men are usually in such a big hurry to remove the thong once they have it in sight that they don't study the fine workmanship, the intricate patterns of the lace, or frankly anything else about this wonderful piece of a woman's arsenal. A woman is just the opposite, taking the time when she purchases the garment to look for all the things that the man later overlooks. Dr. Dog was therefore unprepared for the ferocity of his wife's response, as she said with cold fury, "It's not mine!" Dr. Dog could do no better than turn his head and stare at the thong, still held up with the forceps he had used to remove it from Fluffy, as Mrs. Dog turned on her heel and stormed out the door.

The thong never made it back to its rightful owner. Having made a catastrophic assumption that he knew to whom the garment belonged once, Dr. Dog was at least smart enough not to try to return it to one of the several women who might have been the owner. That's just as well, because Fluffy seems to have a real attachment to the garment, carrying it in his mouth whenever he and the recently divorced Dr. Dog take walks.

A most vexing question presented by this account, all of which was told to me with attestations of its complete veracity, is why Fluffy ate the thong in the first place. Thongs look great, but with rare exceptions, are not made to be eaten. True, Fluffy is a dog, not nearly as smart as most people, and it is possible that he confused the thong for something else. But dogs have sharper senses, and it is highly unlikely that Fluffy's sense of smell would have been fooled into thinking that the thong was something edible.

No, I am convinced that Fluffy ate the thong out of loyalty to Dr. Dog. The dog loved the doctor probably because the doctor was the only one who took Fluffy on really long walks and gave him pigs' ears to eat. When Fluffy came across the thong, lying under the bed in the master bedroom where it had been accidentally kicked in the haste to take it off, he knew that the garment was trouble. It had a very strong scent, different from the subtle scents used by Mrs. Dog. And so, to protect the doctor, Fluffy had eaten the thong as he heard the sound of Mrs. Dog's footsteps approaching.

Cruel irony! Like a real life version of the Gift of the Magi, the dog consumed the thong to protect the doctor only to have the doctor cut the dog open to save the dog, and ruin himself. Like the story, the protagonist's selfless acts made them realize how much they loved each other.

It's a lucky man who has the love of a good dog!

☆ ☆ ☆

My excuse for temporarily putting the spotlight on sex is that God did it first. And it wasn't just the begetting stuff; God at times got very explicit. Take, for example, the awarding to those who kill infidels six dozen virgins with which to entertain themselves. Killing infidels must be way up there in terms of God's priorities because seventy-two virgins, if you think about it, is a heck of a lot of virgins. Thinking through the implications of a 72 -1 ratio led to the following.

Twelfth Interlude:

Dating Advice for Today's Modern Islamic Terrorist

Virtue, some say, is its own reward. When virtue comes at a high price, however, it's comforting to know that God will sweeten the kitty. Take martyrdom, for example. It is always nice to contemplate the death of infidels, but the experience becomes that much richer when one realizes the rewards enjoyed by one who brings about the deaths. I am, of course, talking about spending eternity in the company of seventy-two virgins. Can you imagine the bliss, the ecstasy, of spending eternity in the company of six dozen women, all of whom crave your attention and will do just about anything to get it?

There has been a run on virgins, however, and the stock of available girls was getting too low. Whether owing to the increased number of infidels needing killing, or to the richness of the award, there has been a sharp increase in the number of martyrs blowing themselves up in crowded places. Normally this is not a problem; there is a constant stream of Islamic virgins reaching heaven, and a good many of them are ready to sample the earthly delights they had not enjoyed while alive, once they are assured that it is moral, and that they will be with a proper Islamic hero!

Raise the number of martyrs in any significant way and you see the problem: at a 72-1 ratio, any material increase in the number of martyrs can create shortages in the number of virgins. "We need a solution," God told me privately. "I'd be much obliged if you do a bit of investigation into my options here. Should I reduce the ratio? I mean what man could complain about having 36 women to sleep with? Or I could expand the pool of available women by easing the requirements. Why insist on virginity, when the whole reason for them being here, is, well, you know..." I had the distinct pleasure of looking over my eyeglasses at God, who responded by saying, "Okay smarty-pants. You don't like my ideas? Come back with your own – and let's see who does best."

The first thing I did was to go visit an old friend, Achmed, who had martyred himself ten thousand years ago. It occurred to me as I walked up the street to his house, that I had not seen him for several thousand years. I guessed keeping that many virgins happy kept one busy, and smiled as I rang his doorbell. To my shock, the door opened violently, and a man's naked body hurtled through, nearly knocking me down. As I staggered to keep my balance, I was further amazed to see a "pack" (for there is no other way to describe them) of naked woman who tore after the man. They knocked me down so I didn't actually see the take down of their quarry. But take him down they did, and after some mauling of the poor unfortunate they began carrying him back to the house, all the while keeping up the most lascivious discourse imaginable.

As they passed, I got a good look at the man. It was Achmed. I began to intercede and was ignored, except for one or two death threats. I raised my voice and told them I was on a mission from God, and needed to talk to Achmed. After repeating this several times, I prevailed on them to the extent that they were willing to put him down so we could talk. After that, all bets were off!

"Achmed," I said, "what in heaven's name is going on?"

Instead of answering me, he asked his own question: "Tell me friend, how long is eternity?"

"What?" I said, afraid I had not heard him clearly.

I said, "How long is eternity?"

"Eternity lasts forever," I replied, puzzled by the question.

"Well then, you must tell God that I wish to become a Christian monk. No women! If I have to remain with these women I will go mad!"

"I don't understand," I said, incredulous. "You have it all. You live in splendor with seventy-two beautiful and sexy women. What could be better?"

"You are right, at least for awhile. For the first hundred years it was pure heaven! That one," he said, pointing, "is a gymnast, and that one over there can do things to a man that I still think are impossible." He seemed to get lost in thought, then emerged from his reverie, and said, "Did I say a hundred years? That's unfair. I had real enjoyment for two or three times that long. It's hard to remember exactly how long it took for me to get really sick of the whole thing. Without question, though, by a thousand years, things had gotten old! Little habits of each of the women had begun to grate on me. That one brays like a donkey at the most inappropriate moments; her friend there refuses to kiss on the mouth. At first, these things were mildly annoying, but experience them for thousands of years, and they can make you homicidal! Problem there is that you're not able to kill anyone in heaven. I know; I've tried."

I looked at the women. True, most were disconcerting, undulating their hips and doing all manner of suggestive things. But to try to kill them? I started to think that my former friend was mad.

"I know what you're thinking," he said. "You think I'm nuts." I protested that nothing could be further from the truth. "No I know you do. But that's okay. Listen, do you like a nicely grilled steak?"

This seemed to confirm my earlier diagnosis. But I decided to play along. "I guess I could eat," I responded cautiously.

"No, I don't mean right now. I mean, as a general matter, do you like a grass fed, aged, beautifully marbled, prime rib?"

"As a general matter, yes. You're making me very hungry. What is your point?"

"Don't you see? Imagine that the only food that you could ever eat was prime rib! Imagine that you had it for breakfast, lunch and dinner, for snack, for any reason that you were having food, the only thing that you could eat was prime rib. You'd get pretty sick of it, wouldn't you? Now imagine doing that for year after year after year!" Now, get ridiculous and think in terms of tens of thousands of years!

I was starting to see his point. "So you ceased having sex because you grew tired of it?" I asked.

"It's not that easy," he replied. "I grew sick of it, yes. But I also am surrounded by seventy-two young women who don't look at the world the same way as I do. From their point of view, if I make love to one of them every day, they still only have sex five or six times a year. These are healthy young women, with normal appetites! Try skipping a day, and they attack! Hell, even if I have sex every day some of them still attack. I have become their tool, their pet, forced to do things that make me ill! I tell you, too much of heaven is worse than hell!"

After doing as much as I could to console Achmed, which was precious little, I took my leave of him. The last I saw of him, he was being carried back inside the house while the pack began snarling as to whose turn it was next. The cacophony became so loud that it soon drowned out his whimpers that someone please tell God…

Next I visited Hossein. I expected to find something similar. It was totally different. A chaste young woman, her face concealed, and wearing a garment designed to conceal the curves of her body from strangers, bade us enter. She and the other women looked unspoiled, and exactly how virgins should look.

"Exactly," explained Hossein, when we sat down to talk. "That's because they are still virgins."

"But you've been here for more than a hundred years," I said. "You haven't touched even one?"

"Oh, I've touched them" he said ruefully. "But that's all I can do. You see, I achieved martyrdom by detonating explosives strapped around my waist. In addition to blowing up several infidels, I also blew up my... my equipment!" He started to sob, quietly at first.

"You should ask God," I offered. "Surely He would help."

"You think I didn't?" he cried. "He said that He had better things to do than to reassemble my equipment after I had blown it into a million little pieces. He said I should have thought about what happens to soft tissue when one detonates a bomb six inches away!"

"Tell me about the people you killed with the bomb," I said. "What had they done?"

"Done?" Hossein repeated. "They hadn't done anything that I knew of. But they were non-believers. That's enough!"

Or was it? If God were the father of Islam, Judaism, and Christianity, why would he want members of one of his religions to kill members of the other two? I was so preoccupied with thinking this through that I nearly walked by the address God had given me. It was a charming cottage, surrounded by an even lovelier garden. An older couple was busy tending to an incredible variety of flowers. "Excuse me," I began, "but are the two of you martyrs by any chance?"

"Hmmm. Honey, what do you think?" the man asked his companion. She stopped pulling weeds, and came up to where he was standing.

"Well now, I've never thought about it in those terms," she said. "Tell me, why does it matter?"

"I'm doing some research for God," I explained. "I'm trying to find out whether seventy-two vir…" I caught myself before completing the word, thinking that neither of them would have any notion of what I was doing.

I was wrong. "You were going to say "virgins," weren't you?" The woman asked. "Well, neither of us qualifies, thank God. And I take it that you were wondering whether we qualified for the award of seventy-two virgins, yes?"

I shook my head in the affirmative.

"No dear, heavens no. We were the victims of a bomb blast in the London underground, not the ones who set it off."

I didn't know what to say, and I stammered my apologies.

"Nothing to apologize for," the man said. "You didn't do it. Besides it isn't so bad here. We can grow anything in the garden – it's amazing. And," and here the man looked so lovingly at his companion that I nearly became jealous. "I am with the woman I love through eternity. It's pretty tough to complain, now isn't it?" His eyes belied his words, however, misting as he fought back tears. The woman saw the confusion on my face, and said as she took his hand, "Tut tut. It's okay, luv." Turning to me, she said, "It's our children. They weren't with us when the bomb went off, so they're not here…yet. We miss them terribly."

I took my leave and sat on a park bench to think. I heard a loud "Well?" all around me. I jumped and heard Him chuckle. "God, I hate when you do that," I complained.

"Oh, lighten up," He said, laughing. "If I can't have fun with you, who can I have fun with?" He cocked his head to the side as if in thought. Then he spoke, saying, "You know, I try to use correct grammar. If I didn't who would? But I'll be damned if it sounds better to my ear to say, 'If I can't have fun with you, with whom can I have fun!!?' Sounds to me as if the inmates are in charge of the asylum. Note to self, have that fellow Miriam Webster appear before me first thing in the morning to explain why he shouldn't be some place a bit warmer." Finally, he seemed to remember why he had called me. "Okay, the virgin thing. I assume you have a solution," he said to me.

"The whole virgin thing is a disaster," I said. "The men are miserable. I don't think it is working out as intended."

"Nonsense," God replied. "It is working out exactly as intended. Everything I do works out as I intend. I'm God! You even confirmed a minute ago that the men are miserable."

"Wait, you want the men to be miserable?" I asked.

"Of course," God said, "Otherwise they wouldn't be. I'm God, remember? Look, do you remember the Commandments I issued? Let's see, there were ten of them, with lots of "Thou shalt not..." phrases. Well, one of those phrases was "Thou Shalt Not Kill." Why would I ever reward people who intentionally violate this command!!!??"

His voice rose as he completed that thought. I've been around God for long enough to tell when He was getting worked up – and he was getting worked up! "People think that the manner of their death can make up for a life poorly lived. Why should that be? No, live a miserable life, cause others unhappiness or worse, and think you will escape my wrath? Hah!"

"And another thing. What is this fascination with virgins? If you wanted to play baseball, would you want a pitcher who had never pitched? The truth is that while virginity is attractive for the young, the same condition in a mature woman either means she hasn't been asked, or has persistently turned down the men asking. Now I ask you: why in the world would I give humans a powerful sex drive if I didn't want them to have sex?"

"So you mean," I started, but got no further.

"I mean that these young men who blow people up to please me have shit for brains. I abhor their acts of violence and I abhor their preoccupation with deflowering virgins. If they want to have sex with a virgin, I suggest they try to convince one to do so while they still are alive."

With that, he muttered, "Case Closed," and told me to write it up and distribute it. That is what I've done.

☆ ☆ ☆

I am nervous! Most of you don't know me, and are trying to figure out whether you can relax and trust me. I understand the risks, and do not write about the vagina for prurient reasons. Nor do I write about it lightly. I write about it because it has substantive impacts on our theology that have yet to be realized. For those of you who have not tossed the book already, please give me a chance – this is a serious exposition of religious thought!

THE ORIGINS OF THE VAGINA

Most people start their lives by causing great pain to the women who give them birth. The pain is caused by the mothers-to-be trying to pass their children, including of course their heads, through a passage too small to be well suited for this purpose. Although few would disagree with the statement, no one has pursued the vexing question of why this is. The female body, and more particularly the vagina, works extraordinarily well for the men trying to put something into it, and extremely poorly for the women trying to push something out of it.

This is a major problem for those who believe in intelligent design: either God intended the vagina to be exactly as it is, or He intended it to be different and somehow failed to accomplish what he wanted. If it is as God intended, it doesn't reflect well on God because the design, while great for creating babies, is lousy for delivering them. If it isn't as He intended, that also reflects poorly on God because if He tried to do something better but failed, then He is fallible, and He is not supposed to be. If, as I suspect, He had nothing to do with the design or difficulties of the vagina, then the believers in "Intelligent design" are out to lunch (now there's a surprise), and a woman's body must have reached its present state through means other than God's design. Ironically, evolution is the only explanation that does not require a devaluing of our image of God.

Let's start with the obvious and let logic take us where it will.

Fact: the vagina is extremely well designed for some purposes and poorly designed for others. When it is considered from the man's point of view, it is superbly done. There is no question but that it is engineered to accommodate the man's entry. The vagina is prized, praised and pursued. If there are any complaints at all, it is that men desire to have contact with it far more than they do. It is, in sum, a universal hit with men.

When one considers the vagina's performance as a pathway for delivering a baby, however, few accolades are heard. The design criteria appear unambitious and their implementation sloppy or worse. The standard of performance achieved for its use by men can be described as, "a near perfect experience every time." In contrast, the standard of performance for its use by women during childbirth seems to be that "they should generally but not always survive."

There is no reason why God's design should have been so attentive to the men, and so indifferent to the women. He created huge and complex things that fill us with wonder. He could have designed a channel for delivering babies with a bit more stretch.

Accept as we must that the vagina's design can be approved upon and one must either renounce any involvement in that design by God, or accept that God is either malicious or fallible. Those that seek to hold God responsible for everything run the risk of linking him to much in nature that could be better done.

Those who think more highly of God would do well to consider whether evolution doesn't offer the best explanation of how we got to where we are. It does, though the explanation reveals men to be selfish creatures who don't deserve the love of their mates.

Human beings are only recently civilized. The major part of our history occurred in much rougher times. The choice of sexual partners, unlike now, was largely the prerogative of the male, because he was the stronger physically.

The men at the time were uncomplicated creatures, lacking spirituality. They read little – at most a few cave murals. The men would mate with those women who had attributes that appealed to them, and who made them feel good at the moment. What happened to women nine months from now was not a driver of male behavior. As a result, mutations that would have made for easier deliveries were not selected nor retained in the gene pool; mutations that made the experience more pleasurable for the male were. Modern woman is the result.

I mean no offense to women. This is not a criticism of your bodies, which I can't imagine being more appealing than they are. That is the point – your body is as men would have it; it is women that it sometimes serves less well.

There is no reason to accept the current state of affairs as inevitable. Science has provided us the tools to genetically engineer improved humans. Shouldn't we make improving the birthing experience a key objective for the upcoming century? This is as important as landing a man on the moon.

Just imagine if delivering babies were as enjoyable as making them. Now imagine quintuplets!

As promised, the piece has major theological implications that could not be replicated though use of any other part of the body. What would you do with an elbow, for example?

☆ ☆ ☆

PART IV:

I wrote the following story with my daughter when she was about eight years old. In an attempt to include her in what was otherwise a solitary pastime of mine (writing) I had proposed that we take turns adding a sentence of plot to a story that I would then write in final form. The result was a story called, "My Friend, Oscar." It was the first story I had written for children.

It sat several years in my office, gathering dust. I worked on other projects, including one about the destruction of AT&T, where I had worked for twenty-one years. Frustrated at my inability to get my writing published, I hired an experienced and successful writer to look at the draft AT&T book. That was a big job, which would take some time to start. In the interim, I proposed and she agreed to do a similar job on Oscar.

A few days later, she called with a proposal. She said she loved the Oscar story, and proposed that rather than just edit the story that we become co-authors for that book, and that we do it on a 50-50 basis. I readily agreed, because she had impressed me with her insights and because she was an established writer who had a big-time agent, something I needed and I didn't have.

Artistic differences soon emerged, and my co-author correctly pointed out that one of us had to be the final voice on such decisions. She insisted it be her. At that point, I should have pulled out of the arrangement. I didn't because I wanted to see what would happen if I continued. What happened is that I stopped even getting current drafts before they were shared with her agent and prospective publishers. Virtually every word of the story was changed. The final straw was when the little girl in the story, "Lily," who I had named after my daughter, was renamed "Izzie" because "Lily was too hard for children to pronounce!"

The book was a fine book, but in my opinion, it lacks some of the appeal of the original. I re-print the original story here not to take anything away from the final publication, which I hope you will buy, but as a means of preserving my (and my daughter's) original version of "My Friend, Oscar."

FOURTEENTH INTERLUDE:

MY FRIEND OSCAR

Friends are important. One of my best friends moved away with her parents at the end of first grade. I still miss her a year later. Since I couldn't play with her, I had time to play with other kids I had never played with before. You know what? They're fun too, and now I have more friends than before.

I have one friend that no one can replace. His name is Oscar. I called him Oscar because he is an octopus. You know, Oscar the Octopus. Besides, my name is Lily and "Lily and Oscar" sounded pretty good together. We were friends.

Before you say that would be gross or impossible, let me tell you how it happened. I know it sounds strange. But if you use your imagination, lots of strange things can seem to happen. When I was in first grade, we lived near the shore. Because we were so close to the ocean, we learned a lot about marine life. One day our teacher told us that fish lay thousands and thousands of eggs but that most of them get eaten before they grow up to be adult fish. I remember thinking that was so sad. I wished that one year, the babies would all survive and get to see what it was like to be a grown-up fish. How was I to know that my wish would come true?

The first to notice were the fisherman who came back early with their boats full of fish. None of them could remember a time when the fishing had been so good. Soon there were so many fish that there wasn't room for them all. The ocean was becoming clogged with fish. If you tried to swim, you were likely to end up with at least one or two fish flopping around inside your bathing suit. It got so bad that some of the other marine life left for waters where it was less crowded.

Oscar lived in the waters off the coast of our town. He didn't want to move, but he was getting tired of fish bumping into him while he was trying to sleep. He had seen a large house close to the beach with a large pool beside it, and it looked so inviting. From what he could tell there didn't seem to be any fish in the pool at all. Just a lot of cool, clear water that he could have all to himself!

I know it's pretty unusual for an Octopus to try to cross dry land but that's what Oscar tried to do. He tried to walk the way he had seen the land animals walk, moving one "leg" or in his case "arm" after the other. But an octopus out of the water really can't walk very far. Oscar began getting dizzy, and his arms moved more and more slowly. Then he stopped. It seemed that he wanted to go back to the ocean but was too weak to move.

I had been out with my wagon. I always carried a canteen filled with water with me in case I became thirsty. When I saw Oscar stop, I went up to him, and poured the water over his head. That seemed to help a little bit, and his eyes turned to look at me, but he still wasn't able to move. So as gently as I could, I picked him up and placed him in my wagon. It took a while. Have you ever tried picking up an Octopus? Don't try, because they're not all as friendly as Oscar. But I didn't know that then. Besides, Oscar needed my help.

That was how I rescued Oscar and took him home. We didn't have a pool but we had a big bathtub. Actually, my parents had a big bathtub and I had a small one. I first put Oscar in my bathtub, but I could tell the tub was too small. He could barely move around and his arms—his tentacles— were mostly out of the tub.

I looked down the hallway. No one was there. I put my finger on my lips so that Oscar would know to be quiet. Then I carried him to my parent's bathroom and filled up the tub. That was better. He seemed happier.

I had planned to move him to my bathtub in the morning before my parents woke up. It had been such an exhausting day, though, that I overslept. I would have slept even longer if it hadn't been for the scream that came from my parents' bathroom. My mother had gotten in the tub to take a shower and she and Oscar had met. I didn't know what there was to scream about. My brother had a gerbil, and no one screamed when he ran around on his stupid wheel.

My father had come running. I think they were both a little surprised when I threw my arms around Oscar and told them that he was my pet, Oscar. The best I could do was to get permission for him to stay in my bathtub until the next morning when my father would be able to help return him to the ocean.

The rest of the day, I sat in my bathroom, reading to Oscar and letting him eat all the sardines I had found in the pantry. He tried to eat the soap once, but he didn't like it. Reading always made me a little sleepy, and it had been a pretty exciting morning. But the excitement was just getting started.

Some workmen were building a new garage at a neighbor's house, and one of the men accidentally started an electrical fire. They put it out right away, but the wind carried some sparks to our house, one of which landed in our newspaper pile. The men didn't know that it had happened and went back to work. The papers caught on fire, and the flames started spreading.

My mother was busy putting my brother down for a nap. Oscar really saved the day! He woke me up by tugging at my shirt with his tentacles. As soon as I woke up I smelled smoke. I ran and told my mother, which is what we had always been told to do. Mom took one look at the flames, and took us all outside. Then she ran to a neighbor's house and called the fire department. While she was doing that, I filled up my wagon as high as it would go with water so that Oscar would be comfortable.

You would have to have been there to believe what happened next. The fire truck arrived with only two firemen because they hadn't wanted to wait for the other firemen before coming to our house. It normally takes two firemen to man a fire hose, one to hold it steady and one to aim the hose towards where the water was needed. The firemen had two hoses and they tried to use both but it didn't work. Without someone to hold the hoses down it was really hard to move them around to where they wanted them.

They were about to give up and just use one hose when Oscar crawled out of my wagon, and grabbed hold of the two hoses, holding each with three arms, and grabbing the truck to brace himself with the other two. For a minute, the fireman didn't do anything other than stand staring at Oscar with their mouths open. Then each grabbed a hose, hoping that Oscar would hold it steady. It worked! They put out the fire so quickly that very little was damaged. Oscar held the hoses until the other firemen arrived. He then let go and sank to the ground, tired from being out of the water and working so hard. I gently picked him up and put him back in my water-filled wagon. Even my mother came up to him and patted him on his head. He didn't like that. Somehow I think he and my mother had gotten off on the wrong foot.

Oscar became a hero! The fire department made him their mascot and built a little shelter for him down by the shore.

The generation of fish that had clogged the ocean near us was starting to become a memory. Life went on except that each day I would spend a little time talking to Oscar about the things that were important to me. And do you know what? He sat quietly and would listen to me, without ever interrupting.

I was used to others moving a way. But a few months after I met Oscar, my father told us that he had gotten a better job, and it was our turn to move. He and my mother had talked, and decided that he should take the job. That meant we would be moving too far away for me to see Oscar except during summer vacations. I was sad in the beginning, and spent more time than usual talking to Oscar. I promised him I would come back in the summer to visit him.

I did that first year. I would have come again the following year, but one of the firemen wrote us a letter saying that Oscar had moved as well. The fireman was pretty sure Oscar had swum off to be with other creatures like himself. Maybe he even has a family of his own!

I miss Oscar. Who wouldn't? But it doesn't make me sad any more. I knew that Oscar really wouldn't have been happy living in a bathtub, and I couldn't have lived in the ocean. Somewhere out there, though, I have a friend with eight arms. Now how many people can say that? My dad says if I can hold on to my imagination as I grow up, Oscar and I will probably run into each other again. I can't wait.

☆ ☆ ☆

I wrote a second Oscar story. Because in the published Oscar story, Lily didn't move away, the perceptive among you will notice that this story assumes that she hadn't moved either. Because the first Oscar book didn't sell well, no one was interested in publishing a sequel. Here it is.

Oscar swam slowly, feeling very sorry for himself. The pool where he had worked as a lifeguard had closed at the end of summer, and he had come back to the ocean. Oh, he had tried living with the little girl again. He liked her. But the little girl's mother made him nervous, and being nervous got him into trouble.

The little girl had been explaining something or other to Oscar, using those funny sounds that she made. Oscar didn't understand a single word she was saying, although he was pretty sure that when she said "Oscar" she meant him. He guessed this because she would say "Oscar" and then poke him. After a dozen pokes, he decided the sound meant either him, or "to annoy." But she also said "Oscar" upon seeing him, without poking him at all, so he decided the sound meant him. He also decided that her name was "Lily," because she pretended to poke herself while saying, "Lily."

Oscar's other guesses about what Lily said were not very good.

Because Lily talked a lot about her mom in advising Oscar how to behave, he naturally assumed the sound "mom," meant "fish," the most common word in conversations among octopuses. To make matters worse, Oscar decided that "mom" didn't mean just any fish. Judging by the concern in Lily's voice when she tried telling Oscar about how to behave around her "mom," Oscar guessed that "mom" meant a big, scary fish. Maybe even a shark!

Now Oscar could protect himself against sharks. But they still made him nervous. So when Lily approached her mother, and said,

"Mom, I promise it will be different this time. Can Oscar stay? Please mom! Please mom! Puh-leeeese," Oscar heard only his name, then a bunch of meaningless sounds, and then "scary fish! Scary fish!"

Now Oscar was as brave as the next Octopus, but his natural instinct when afraid was to squirt ink and run for cover, and that is what he did. All over her mother. And the kitchen cabinets. And the dishes that her mom had just washed that were neatly stacked next to the sink.

"Oh, Oscar," Lily said. She looked at her mom, the ink slowly dripping from her hair onto her face, and then onto the nice white collar of her blouse, and said, "C'mon Oscar, I'll take you back to the ocean now."

Now, two days later, Oscar was swimming without knowing where he should go. He missed the little girl a lot, and not only because she gave him those shiny little boxes stuffed with lots of headless little fish. He missed her too because she had made all sorts of noises at him, called him Oscar, and patted his arms while saying things like, "I love you, Oscar." (This last thing, Oscar assumed – like almost everything else, based on the warmth in the little girl's eyes when she said it, that she meant, "Would you like some fish to eat?)

So far as we know, octopuses don't smile when they're happy. But if they do, Oscar did. Something had clicked in his brain, and he decided to go back, at least for a visit.

Oscar swam to where he used to sit on some large rocks piled near the shore. It had been a favorite spot of Lily's where she would talk things out with herself, with Oscar listening, when she was upset.

She was there talking to herself. "What a stupid time to have a talent show," she fumed. "I mean, why pick now to have one, and why have a whole section on stupid pets? Boy, I wish Oscar were here. I'd show them a thing or two!"

Oscar smacked the water with one of his arms and caught her attention. "Oscar!" she shrieked. "Where did you come from? Oh, it doesn't matter. I'm just glad that you're here." Lily gave Oscar a hug, and then got serious. "Oscar, I need your help for the talent show. Can you catch?"

She spent the next half hour throwing various things at Oscar. He made no effort to catch them – sometimes balls would bounce right off him. Lily sighed. The talent show was tomorrow and she didn't know what to do.

A bully named Roscoe made things worse, if that were possible. He snickered upon hearing that Lily was going to have an Octopus perform with her. "Yeah, right, loser!" he said. "A trained Octopus? You're crazy!" To make certain that his view was not misunderstood, he pushed Lily to the ground and walked away.

"We'll show him," the little girl said, throwing a ball to Oscar. It fell harmlessly among his many arms.

It was her mom that offered the solution, asking whether Lily had tried throwing something Oscar liked, like fish. "Sardines!" Lily exclaimed. She ran to the kitchen, came back with the three cans of sardines that she found, and threw one to Oscar.

Thwack! Oscar neatly caught it with one of his tentacles, and then used his suction cups to tear it open, consuming the little fish inside.

"It works, it works," she said, excitedly. "It's Thursday, It's Thursday," Oscar decided she meant, for no very good reason at all.

The next day at the talent show, Oscar repeated his perfect performance, catching all six cans of sardines Lily threw to him. He ate three of them. He wanted to eat the others too, but he didn't. Instead, Oscar threw one of them for a perfect strike, hitting the bully right on his bottom!

"Ow!" Roscoe said. "Hey, who did that?" He looked around angrily, and saw Oscar holding the other two cans. For a moment, he tried to look tough. Then his lip quivered, and he started crying. Like most bullies, he was afraid to confront an angry octopus. Especially one armed with sardine cans.

What's more to say? Lily and Oscar won the talent show, and Oscar got to eat the cans of sardines he hadn't already eaten. Lily gave him a hug, which he really enjoyed. He just wished she hadn't seen her mom approach and said in the middle of the hug, "Thanks, scary fish!" That made him nervous, and when he got nervous, he....

Squirt!

☆☆☆

As Lily grew older, the stories adapted. We used to take walks together, and the next story was based on a conversation we had during one of those walks.

JUST BEFORE THE SNOW

Have you ever imagined that it snowed so much that it covered all the doors and windows? I mean, even the windows of the bedrooms on the second floor? Lily not only imagined it; she was deeply troubled by it. How would they get food to eat? How would they ever get out of the house?

She decided that the matter was serious enough to discuss with her father, who at first tried to avoid the topic which such parental favorites as "It will never happen," or "Isn't this something you would prefer to discuss with your mother?" Finally, having headed off every dodge, she saw her father grow thoughtful. You might wonder how she knew. It was easy: when she forced him to think, she noticed that he almost always tilted his head a little to the left and squinted his eyes, so that wrinkles appeared on his forehead.

"So how would we eat?" she demanded.

"Are you kidding?" he replied. "You always make fun of me for keeping so much pasta in the cupboard. I figure that if you didn't get tired of pasta, we would be able to last through at least two or three seasons before we ran out. By then the snow would melt and we could get out."

"But, how are you going to cook the pasta," she asked. "With a snow like this, the power will go off. It always does. That means no water, and no electricity." She thought she had him now. Her logic was correct. We had a well, with the water brought from the well to the house by an electric pump. No electricity; no pump; no pump, no water.

"Well, the water is kind of easy," he started. "I would just go up to the second floor, open a window and scoop a bunch of snow and put it into a pot. Water would not be a problem."

"But electricity would be," she pounced. She smiled confidently and was about to tell him that they would all starve to death because of his lack of imagination!

He gave a little smile, and said, in violation of every rule she could think of, that he would use an oil generator he kept in the garage for just such an occasion.

"What oil generator?" she asked. "When did you get it?"

"Just before the snow," he began, "I sniffed the air and thought it smelled like snow. So I bought a generator just before the snow started."

"Da-a-ad," she said, "you can't do that. I mean, even if you had bought a generator, you'd still run out of oil to run it."

"Well, I might have but just before the snow, after I had sniffed the air and smelled snow and bought the generator, I thought to myself that a generator isn't much good without fuel. So I had two large underground tanks installed, each one holding five hundred gallons. And I had both tanks set up to automatically feed the fuel into the generator when I push a button. The man who set it up said it would last at least three seasons."

"Da-a-a-ad!" the girl shrieked. "You can't just make stuff up that doesn't make any sense. It would take way too much time to install those tanks. You wouldn't have had the time to do it. There wasn't much time between the time you smelled the snowstorm, assuming you did, and the storm itself. Putting two huge tanks in the ground would have taken weeks! No way. We are going to starve to death."

The father thought for a moment, and said, "That's very good, Lily. You would have been right, except…" he paused for effect, prompting Lily to interrupt.

"Except…" she said.

"Except, just before the snow, I had invented a time machine. Which I did. You see, after I smelled the snow and bought the generator I knew I wanted to install fuel tanks. But I knew that there wouldn't be enough time to get it done before the storm hit. So I built a time machine, went back three months, and ordered the tanks. Would you believe it, the company that does it was so busy with winter coming that I decided to go back to last summer. I was lucky; they were having an off-season sale."

There was never a little girl who wanted to starve as much as Lily, it seems. She thumped her feet on the ground, saying, "Dad, it is impossible to travel through time. Besides, even if it were possible for some braniac to figure it out, you wouldn't be the one person to figure out how to do it. You always have told me that you weren't that good at science."

"That normally would be true," he responded. "Except for one thing. I really stumbled upon how to travel through time by accident. It was only after I could travel in that way that I decided, just before the snow, that I ought to travel back a few years and study everything I could about time. So I got a doctorate in Physics at Princeton University. That education then helped me stumble onto the concept of space travel years later when I would need it. It's amazing, frankly, how close Albert Einstein came to getting it all right. You know who he is, right? He's just about the smartest person who ever lived and he taught at Princeton the last years of his life, trying to figure out time. I just tweaked one of his equations and poof! I understood how to take advantage of time's imperfections."

"Excuse me?" Lily said, looking dubiously at her father.

"I presume you've heard about $E=mc^2$?" He looked at her blank expression and decided he could risk it, concluding, "That is so close! But it doesn't really work. It should have been $E=mc^2$-27. It's an incredibly small error when you consider the size of the other numbers but it throws it off just enough to make his equation unusable."

Lily could only look at her father who was smiling back at her. She inhaled deeply and sighed. Then she said, "Dad, have you ever imagined that it became so hot that you couldn't leave the house because the soles of your shoes would melt before you had taken two steps. And we were stranded in our house and there was no water anywhere to drink or cook pasta or…"

Her dad looked beaten. Then, however, he said, "That sounds like there is no way out. And there wouldn't have been, except that, just before the heat wave…"

And so they went on hour after hour, enjoying life in very boring weather that was neither a blizzard nor a heat wave, but imagining what they would do in the very worst of circumstances.

☆☆☆

This next story is the last "children's" story to make the cut. I remember reading this story to Lily for the first time. We were on the Amtrak train, heading south from Boston to our home in New Jersey, or at least as close to home as Amtrak will get you. We were supposed to get off at Metropark, which is about a 45-minute drive from where we lived.

Anyway, about twenty minutes from our destination, I asked my daughter whether she wanted to hear my latest story. She said yes, and we began. We became engrossed in the story and missed our station. The next stop was Trenton, which was more than a half hour away. We had no choice but to ride to Trenton, and then get off, wait for a northbound train, and go back. My advice would be to not begin this story while cooking, or frankly, doing anything that requires your presence in the immediate future.

Seventeenth Interlude:

The Magical Odds and Ends Store

Chapter One

The store was there before the neighborhood. It was old, not quite as old as the old man who owned it and was the sole employee, but it had to be fifty years old at least. Lily knew it was at least that old because like many old buildings, it had the year carved right into one of the foundation stones. "1955," it read. It had a window display, in which a sign still appeared advertising milkshakes, though Lily had learned from experience that they hadn't served those in years.

The window was dirty with years of deposits from the city air. You could just see the fantastic clutter of dusty old things that made the store seem like a giant attic, filled with all sorts of things that were nearly wonderful, except for some minor problem that made you want to keep them, but just not use them every day. And as long as Lily could remember, the same sign made of neon that no longer lit hung above the doorway, one of those signs that were hung on brackets so that it was perpendicular to the store. The sign said simply "MOES."

The neighborhood had been started in the 1960's and now every usable lot had a home on it. It wasn't exactly a suburb, being too close to the city center to allow huge yards, with acres and acres of grass. But there were neat town homes with small yards. You can tell a lot by looking at the cars in driveways – here, there were lots of new or almost new cars, not particularly fancy but not the bottom of the heap, either. The people who lived there were not rich, but they were comfortable. They had jobs and they had some extra money to spend every month.

The store didn't belong. Lily's parents weren't different than most: they saw no reason to go into the "filthy old store" themselves, and they certainly didn't want their children to go into such a place without them. As a result, the store seemed to do very little business. There were only a handful of regular customers that seemed to frequent it. Most of these seemed very rich, with big limousines dropping them off and picking them up right in front of the store.

Lily never would have gone in there, except for the scavenger hunt. Lily was ten now, a year older than her friend Victoria. The two had met when Lily, who stayed with her father in the neighborhood on weekends, had tried to make money selling hot chocolate in her father's driveway. Lily had not sold enough to break even, but one of her customers had been Victoria. The two had become fast friends. When Victoria had shown Lily a flyer about a month-long scavenger hunt, which advertised that contestants would be challenged to find the most unusual and fantastic things, and that the grand prize would be a family vacation in Italy, the two girls decided to enter. The only problem was that in order to enter, you needed a hundred dollars, and you needed to submit the first item on the scavenger contest list.

"Which is?" asked Lily.

'It says you are to bring in an actual sign from a gas station," Victoria replied. She paused, reading on and then added, "Oh my, that's really hard."

"What? Tell me," Lily said, eager with the anticipation of some impossible condition.

"It says that the sign must say that gasoline costs twenty-seven cents a gallon." She looked up at Lily, and asked, "Did gasoline ever cost only twenty-seven cents a gallon?"

Lily thought for a moment before saying, "I don't know. I know it's a few dollars a gallon now. That seems really, really cheap. Maybe a long time ago… Let's go ask someone old like my dad. He'll know!"

The two girls found Lily's father, who felt rather good that day for someone so old. But he was old, I guess, because he remembered when gasoline cost twenty-seven cents a gallon. "Not only did it cost about that, but they also gave you a free glass, kind of nice actually, to entice you to fill up at their gas station rather than someone else's," he added.

They didn't care about the glass. "But where can we find a sign from, what did you say, the 'fifties or sixties'?" Victoria asked.

"Dang if I know," Lily's father responded, "I think that it will be next to impossible." He saw their crestfallen looks, and then added, "Why don't you try Moe's? Who knows; that might be just the sort of thing he sells in there."

Because neither girl was supposed to go into the store without a parent, and no parent had ever wanted to go there before, this was both Lily's and Victoria's first time in the store. Well, it was actually Lily's second time, if you were to count that time that, against her parents' more or less clear instructions, she poked her head inside to see if they made milk shakes. But that didn't officially happen and besides she hadn't really looked around, so we will not count it here. Officially.

Both girls stared with their eyes as big as saucers the moment they went in and this time, did look around. Unlike the outside of the store, which made you not want to enter, the inside was bright and cheery, with interesting things everywhere you looked. There were two horses from an old merry-go-round, shiny jewelry, swords that looked real, and this and that and the other thing. There was also a fire in the fireplace, a real one that helped tame the November chill in the air.

Lily's father summed up all of their reactions the way an adult with advanced college degrees would. "Wow," he said. The girls answered the way a child who had yet to go to college would. "Double wow," said Victoria. "Double wow plus one," said Lily.

As they stared with open mouths at the wondrous display of totally unnecessary things, Victoria happened to notice the old man sitting with his head down, looking very much like he was sleeping in his chair by the fireplace. She called her companions attention to him, and Lily walked over and looked more closely at him. He had a kindly face, one of those whose lines had been etched by laughter. On top of his head, there was not a single hair, save for little grey tufts around the ears.

Lily drew close enough so that had she reached out she could have touched the man. She thought about doing so, but jumped back in fright as the man, his head still down, asked in a voice way too loud to come from someone sleeping, "May I help you, young lady?"

None of them spoke for a moment, so startled were they. The father then, having his wits about him a bit more than the two girls, said, "Good morning. Listen, the girls here – that one is Lily, my daughter, and this is Victoria, her friend – wanted to participate in a scavenger hunt and they need to find a gas station sign showing the price for gasoline to be only twenty-seven cents per gallon. Do you have that sort of thing?"

"A scavenger hunt, eh?" the old man said. "What fun, what fun." He then stared off in space, looking like he was remembering something, before adding, one last "what fun."

Lily brought things into focus by saying, "Well do you?"

The man now looked at Lily, furrowed his brow, and said, "Do I what?" Lily felt a wave of sympathy for the poor, confused old man. She went up to him, leaned over for the man was still in his chair, and gave him a soft kiss on his cheek. She then spoke to her father and Victoria, saying, "We'd best be going." And finally, she turned towards the door, telling the old man, "Thanks very much. We'll let you know if we find one."

As Lily reached the door, the old man spoke, this time in a clear, strong voice. "Hmmmm, the request is most unusual. You said twenty-seven cents, even. But gas stations have a practice, they have for years, of rarely if ever charging an even number of cents per gallon. Have you noticed? They always add nine tenths of a cent after a number. They can't resist trying to fool the public into thinking that a last tenth of a cent knocked off the price makes it cheaper."

"So what do you think they want? Do they want a sign that says twenty-seven and nine tenths cents or do they perhaps want twenty-six and nine tenths of a cent, that being closer to twenty-seven cents than the other?"

Victoria was the first to recover the shock of the man suddenly speaking, and looked at the flyer announcing a scavenger hunt and said, "I don't know; it just says twenty-seven cents." Lily just stared at the man, a smile beginning to appear on her face. She added to what her friend Victoria had said, saying, "You are going to help us aren't you?"

"We'll just have to see about that. Finding such things can be expensive, you know," the old man said.

"Now look here," Lily's father said. "Do you have such a sign or not?

It's hardly worth discussing price if you don't. And if you do, I am sure we could work out a reasonable price." He emphasized the word reasonable as he said this, stretching it out as if each letter was a half note in four-four time.

The old man replied, "Oh I have one, or I can get it. But you see the problem may be that I want unreasonable compensation for it." He took an old jar and with another smile, turned to Lily and asked, "Have you ever caught fireflies?"

"Sure," Lily answered. "Lots of times."

"Well, don't. It's cruel to them. But I want you to do something very similar. I want you to catch the sun's first rays tomorrow morning. Open the jar just as the sun comes up. Wait about a minute. Then put the lid on and bring it to me. Do you think you can do that?"

"Yes," answered Lily who thought of saying all sorts of things like "But you can't catch sunlight in a jar," but thought better of saying them.

"Great. Now let me see about that gas station sign," the old man said. He held up his finger as if to say "just a minute" and went through a door into a storage area in the back of the store. He poked his head out in a minute, and added, "Now no peeking!" Then he disappeared again, this time solidly shutting the door behind him.

Almost immediately, brilliant white light streamed under the door, as if an explosion of light had occurred in the storeroom. But before any of them had time to say anything, the light was gone and the old man reappeared, carrying three bulky signs. "Give me a hand, will you," he said to Lily's father. As he handed the first of the signs to him, he explained, "I really didn't want to guess which sign they wanted, so I got all three. This one is for gas, priced at twenty-seven point nine cents," and he handed the sign to Lily's dad. "This one is for twenty-six point nine cents," and he handed the second one over. Then he took a smallish sign, and almost reverently handed it to Lily's father. "And this one is a real rarity, advertising gasoline for twenty-seven cents even. There was a small family run gas station outside of Chicago that always priced its gas without any nonsense like the nine tenths of a cent. This was a sign they used in 1950."

Again, the three visitors stood, open mouthed, gaping in wonder. "But how did you find all these things?" asked Lily's father.

The old man looked puzzled by the question. "Now where would you think you'd find a gas station sign? At a gas station, of course."

"But…" Lily's father began, before a look from Lily made him decide not to press the point. Instead, he said, "I can't thank you enough, Mr. …" he paused realizing he didn't know the old man's name. "Is it Mr. Moe, or is Moe your first name?" he asked.

"Heavens, no," said the old man. "My friends call me Curly," came the response. "Curly" ran his hand over his bald head as he said this.

Lily's father said, "I get it. Is that where the name "Moe" comes from too?" He happened to look over at the two girls as he asked this and they both were looking at him strangely, so he explained, "Look, it's way before your time but there used to be a comedy group called "The Three Stooges." Their names were Curly, Moe and Larry. Is that where the names are from?"

The old man looked puzzled. "The three who?" he asked. "No, he continued, my late wife started calling me Curly when I lost my hair. Every time someone calls me Curly it reminds me of her. So that's what I'd like you to call me. As for the name MOES isn't a name for anyone. It describes this store, I think. It stands for the "Magical Odds and Ends Store. As you've already seen."

Lily's dad frowned a bit. "It is pretty amazing that you had the signs," he said, "but I don't want the girls to think that it is 'magic.' You know I am trying to root them in science."

"Of course," Curly responded, "Good thinking. The only thing is that it IS magic, and it IS completely scientific. Magic is just the name we give to science that we don't yet understand." And with that he went off humming, leaving Lily's dad to wonder what he meant.

Chapter Two

The day by which entrants had to submit their entries to the scavenger hunt was the following Saturday. Even though they had the sign, they also needed to raise the one hundred dollar entrance fee. They started with forty-two dollars at the beginning of the week, and by doing every errand and extra chore they could think of during the week they built that up to eighty dollars by Saturday morning. They didn't know how they were going to raise the last twenty dollars, when their two fathers came up to them. Victoria's father spoke first, saying, "You know, if you win this contest the prize you win is a trip for a family of four. What do you say we do a double father-daughter thing? If you are willing, it's worth the extra twenty dollars."

This caused a round of hugs and kisses as both daughters expressed their thanks. Lily's dad then said, "C'mon, we need to get going. The rules say that contestants must present the sign by three p.m. We'll make it without problem, but we ought to get going." They made it with plenty of time to spare, even after spending a long time looking for parking. They finally parked in an expensive parking lot, for which Lily's dad paid. The happy girl told him that she loved him, to which he responded that "he was just protecting his investment."

Once inside, it was surprisingly not a mob scene. Oh, there were plenty of people who were involved in running the scavenger hunt, and there were even people who were curious about the thing that they were there simply as spectators. But there were a surprising absence of other contestants. In fact there was only one other group.

You could tell immediately that they were contestants by the suspicious and unfriendly looks they gave everyone new who walked into the room. They were extremely well dressed, and Lily guessed that they belonged to the stretch limo they had seen parked in a no-parking zone right out front. As the two girls approached the check-in desk with their signs, two from the group who seemed in charge walked over to intercept them. "Oh really, now, George," said the woman to the man, "do you think that these juveniles will really have followed directions when no one else has seemed to? I mean, girls," and she turned to Lily and Victoria now with a put-on sweet smile, "did you know that the requirement is for twenty-seven cents even, without any of those silly nine-tenths tacked on.

The woman obviously expected her news to crush the girls. Lily just gave a big grin and the two of them continued to walk to the check-in desk. You could tell that the people there were fed up with George and Priscilla (for that was the name of the woman who had spoken), and were hoping that at least one other contestant would qualify. It was a young man who spoke to them, saying, "Yes it's true. We made a mistake in the flier announcing the contest, and now these two look like they are going to be the only ones to qualify." He then leaned closer and lowered his voice, finishing, "Although if you ask me, I think their sign is a fake. If you look closely it seems like there was a "nine" after the twenty-seven. But this a charity event, and we are not prepared to fight that in court, which those two threatened us with."

The young man was handsome, and looked to be the right age to be in college. Both girls had this dreamy look as they listened to him, and neither of them spoke when he stopped. It was Lily's dad who broke the spell. "Listen, young man, I don't know about their sign but we have a genuine sign for twenty-seven cents. In fact, we didn't know which one you wanted so that we brought one of each price – twenty-seven even, twenty-six point nine and twenty-seven point nine."

There was a lot of activity at the desk now, as the young man looked at the sign and then announced that it met the requirements and they were officially entered into the scavenger hunt! This brought a mini-celebration of all those there except of course George and Priscilla. The two of them looked at the girls with great hostility, asking them where they got "this sign that you say is genuine." They were about to answer when both fathers jumped in telling the nasty twosome that that was a professional secret.

About the same time, the young man who had taken their submission said in a loud voice, "May I have your attention please. We are in the unexpected situation of having only two teams qualify. But as the Smiths here (and here he looked at Priscilla and George) told me, the contest must go on. We will however, in light of the small number of contestants involved, reduce the number of rounds to two – that is the contest will be decided by who finds two items, one easy and one almost impossibly difficult." Priscilla started to object to something but as she opened her mouth to do so, the young man added, "Of course, you will find the authority to reduce the number of rounds in your rules, specifically Rule 11.2" He had guessed right; Priscilla closed her mouth and said nothing.

George yelled out, "That's Smythe, not Smith," but otherwise raised no complaint.

The young man spoke again, "Of course, Mr. Smy-y-y-the," he said drawing out his corrected use of their name. "The Smythes and our young friends," and here he winked at the two girls will need to find first a rare coin, a Lincoln penny, dated 1909 with an "S" on it marking its manufacture at the San Francisco mint, and with the initials of the penny's designer, Victor D. Brenner, or "VDB" on the back side of the coin. One caveat, the coin must be found by the team; it cannot be purchased. You have one week."

Lily's dad gave a whistle, "Boy oh boy," he said. "I collected Lincoln pennies when I was a kid, fifty years ago. I remember even then, and I am talking about a time a heck of a lot closer to 1909 than now. This was the one penny I never found. Guys, you can try going through rolls of pennies but unless you could buy it somewhere, which you can't and I couldn't afford, I just think it's a real long shot to find this."

Lily turned to the young man who had identified the coin as their target. She asked him, "Excuse me, I'm just wondering. You said that there was going to be one easy thing to find and one hard one. Which one is this?"

The young man gave her a sympathetic look. Then he replied, "This one is the easy one."

Chapter Three

On their way home, Lily, Victoria and their respective fathers stopped at a bank. They went in and each of the fathers gave the girls an "advance" of twenty dollars. Then the girls took the combined forty dollars up to the teller and asked for pennies. The teller didn't have that many and asked if they really wanted that many pennies. "Of course," said Lily who was still trying to figure out exactly how many that would be. The first teller then went to the other tellers and together they amassed a pile of rolls of pennies.

"There you are," he said, and then he and Lily said at the same time (for she had just figured it out), "four thousand pennies!" That seemed like a lot; it was a lot. Pennies came in rolls of fifty, so they had eighty rolls! At home, the girls were filled with optimism as they poured them into a mountain and begin sifting through them, putting the pennies that were not from 1909 back into rolls. The optimism faded as the work continued. Victoria did find a penny from 1917 but that was the closet any of them got. They finished shortly before dinner. Lily's eyes were welling up with tears of frustration, so her father tried to make her feel better by saying that they could take these pennies to other banks, exchange them and try again.

"Realistically, dad, what are our chances?" Lily asked.

"Not good," he answered, "but that is no reason to give up!"

"Maybe tomorrow. Dad." Lily said. "Right now, I've got to go pay Curly for the sign." As she said his name, she couldn't prevent a little smile. It lightened her mood. She took the bottle that she had used to capture the light and went to see Curly.

He was sitting in the same chair, with his head down, but this time Lily spoke to him as soon as she entered. "Well, Curly, your sign worked. Thank you so much. I brought the jar which I caught the first rays of the sun yesterday, but…"

When he heard her mention the jar, he perked up, looking up and giving her a big smile. "Thank you, thank you, thank you," he said. "So how are you going to find the penny? It is extraordinarily rare you know."

"But how did you know?" she asked.

"Tut, tut, child," he replied. "I heard about it on the radio. You are famous, you know. They had an interview with the company sponsoring the contest. They're very disappointed that the mistake about the sign has limited the number of contestants to only two. At least they were at first. Now they are warming up to the idea, because the fact that there are only two is generating all sorts of interests in the event. You know, the rich obnoxious couple versus the pretty young girls. Might versus right, so to speak."

He was grinning as she looked at him. "Well, I am afraid the contest isn't going to last much longer," she said. "I don't think we are going to find the penny. I don't know if the Smythes will either since they won't be able to buy it this time."

"Oh but they already have," he said. "You haven't been listening to the news, I take it."

"No, I haven't," she said. "But the rules say that they can't buy it. Right?"

"Right!" he said. "But the problem with rules is that there are always people who find some way to get around them. They didn't buy the coin, which was all the rule prohibited. They bought a coin store that happened to have the coin in its inventory."

"Can they do that?" she asked, starting to twirl her hair with her fingers.

"They did, and I would guess that they will get away with it," he replied. "Life isn't always fair," he added, seeing the tears welling up in the corners of her eyes. He stared at her for a minute and then said, "Look, I happen to have such a coin. It is yours as a gift, but I do want something in return."

As she heard him say he had the coin, she threw her arms around him in a spontaneous display of affection. "You are the best, Curly! I don't know how I am ever going to thank you enough."

He blushed from the attention, and said, "Yes, well, ahem, I mean, you have got to give me something too. You know what I want? I love fireworks. I want a painting or photograph, your choice, of a fireworks display. Not just any fireworks display, though. It has to have red, lots of beautiful red. Can you do that for me?"

She gave him a puzzled look, but said, "Of course I can. Is that all you want?"

"Is that all?" he said, repeating the question. "My gosh, but that is exactly what I want."

"Okay, you've got it," she said. She made arrangements to come back on Friday, the day before the week was up, to see him about the coin. In the meantime, she caught up with the news. The Smythes had indeed bought a coin store, and it had been ruled legal by a judge. The young man had called Lily's father and had told him, asking how their search was going. Lily had not shared with anyone that Curly had the coin, and her father was unaware of it. He answered, putting on a brave front, but it was hard to keep the pessimism out of his voice. "We have gone through the pennies at six different banks so far, totaling about twenty-four thousand pennies. No luck yet, but we're going to keep trying."

"Well, good luck," the young man said, I guess it doesn't hurt to tell you that we are all pulling for the girls to win. Tell them to keep their spirits up!"

Lily was going to tell her father about the coin, but decided to keep it as a surprise instead. The only one she shared it with was Victoria, and they had a real giggle-fest that neither father could understand. The men were even more confused when they suggested going to go to a new bank, and were told by Victoria that the girls were too busy just then! Nor did it become any clearer when the two girls started painting pictures of a firework display. Victoria's father rolled his eyes, commenting that there was no understanding this new generation of kids.

Friday arrived and the two girls went to present their fireworks picture to Curly. He looked at it, and – as he almost always seemed to be doing – smiled. "Thank you again," he said, a bit of a tear forming in one eye.

Victoria noticed, and asked, "Is everything okay? Is the picture what you wanted?"

"Never better," came his response. "Yes, the picture is exactly what I wanted." He then took from underneath his counter a small envelope, continuing, "I think you will find the item inside of some interest."

Victoria opened the envelope. Inside was another plastic envelope, and inside and clearly visible was a coin. On its face was the year 1909 and underneath the date was the letter "s". That was it. Victoria had a momentary panic, until Lily whispered, "No, I think the other letters are on the other side." Victoria looked, and on the bottom of the back of the coin were the initials "VDB."

Neither girl had collected coins before but the knowledge that they were looking at something so old and so rare still affected them. "Wow," said Lily. "Double-wow," said Victoria. "Plus one," said Lily.

Thanks were handed around, and then the girls returned to their homes. Lily's father was waiting. He gave her a sympathetic look, before saying, "Lily, tomorrow is the day the pennies are due. I wish this weren't happening because it's a horrible lesson for you to learn, but..."

Lily interrupted. "Dad," she said, "It's okay. Really."

"My little girl is growing up," her father said proudly.

"Yes, I am," she replied, a little bit of exasperation showing in her voice. "But it's okay because we..." Lily paused for effect and then remembered that Curly had wanted them to wait until the last minute to reveal they had the coin. "Out of an abundance of caution," he had said. "I just don't want the Smythes to know that you have anything." He had also told her to keep the real coin in her pocket while wrapping up a regular penny in the envelope that she would carry. "Just on a hunch," he had added.

"Well, you'll see dad, it will be okay," Lily said.

A few hours later they were back downtown at the hunt headquarters. The Smythes had presented their coin already, and had approached them as they entered the building. "Are you here to throw in the towel," Priscilla asked?

"Listen, you…" Lily's dad began, his voice a bit heated.

Lily interrupted. "It's okay, dad, we have it," she said.

Lily's dad and Priscilla both said at the same time, "What did you say?"

"I said that we have the coin for the scavenger hunt," Lily said. Lily couldn't be certain but thought she saw Priscilla look at a man hanging back in the shadows. But, as Lily said that she had the coin, the man started running towards them. Before she or anyone else could react, he snatched the envelope she had waved when she spoke from her hand, and continued running. There were two policemen by the door but they too were taken by surprise and before they could react the thief had burst through the door. Though they pursued him they could not catch him. He and the envelope were gone.

Priscilla yelled weakly, "Stop thief," before turning to Lily and saying, "You poor dear, perhaps you can ask the judges whether they can grant some small delay to enable you to try to get your coin back," she said, her voice oozing with false compassion. Of course, she already knew the answer about the delay. She had told the judges this morning that she would oppose any such delay, after they had explained that if one party objected, there could be no delay.

Lily looked at Priscilla with a look of utter distaste. She bit her lip for a moment, suppressing what she wanted to say, and then said, "No need to worry. I had a good friend who warned me that something might happen, and so I carried the penny in my pocket. At this, Priscilla's face changed. Starting with a very false smile, her face moved through a phase of reddened anger to an almost white fury. With her fingers pulled into tight fists, she managed to say through clenched teeth, "how very lucky."

Lily walked up to the desk, pulled her hand out of her pocket, and gave the young man a coin. He looked at the front of it, then the back of it, and said into the microphone, "Ladies and gentlemen, it is a 1909 Lincoln penny, made in San Francisco, bearing the initials VDB on the back. We are on to the third and final round!"

Chapter Four

The young man cleared his voice and proceeded. "This next round is going to be tough. The object of this hunt is music. Not just any music; we are looking for previously unknown and unpublished work of a major composer. It can be of any composer that the judges view as significant. The decision of whether the composer is significant will be made by the judges and is in their sole discretion. Should you each find music meeting the description the winner will be decided upon which composer and which piece the judges view as being the most significant and relevant. Again, the judges' decision on these issues is in their sole discretion. Their decisions are final and may not be challenged.

Lily's dad whistled. "Wow," he said. "Double-wow," said his daughter. "Double-wow plus one," said Victoria.

"They weren't kidding about this one being difficult," Victoria's father added, "How does one find previously unpublished music?"

"Well," said Lily's father, "one way is to pay some musician to write something new. You can bet that is what the Smythes will do."

Lily realized her dad was correct, but did not panic. Thus far, Curly had been more than a match for the Smythes and their money. She asked her dad if they could stop in to see him on their way home. After conferring with Victoria's dad, he said yes.

He was in his usual position, sitting head down on the chair by the fire. Lily had learned his habits well enough so that she began speaking immediately. "Curly," she said, "You are a genius. Someone did try to steal the coin you gave me. By keeping it in my pocket as you suggested, they were unable to. We're in the last round."

"I know," he said. "Congratulations." Then, not waiting to be asked, he said, "And I presume you want to know what kind of undiscovered music I keep in stock. The answer is not very much and nothing certain to win. But," and here he paused until they could barely stand the suspense.

"But what…" Victoria finally prompted.

"But I could get something certain to win," Curly said, and then with a wink, "But this time you've got to earn it."

"I don't understand," Lily said, "how could we possibly earn enough to pay for an…" She thought a minute, and then added, "I suppose if we got something old that had never been seen before…" She thought some more, and then said, "Like the Beatles!"

"I'm thinking older," Curly said, and then he paused for what seemed like forever to hook his audience, before concluding, "like Beethoven!"

At first no one was amazed because no one took Curly seriously. But he was so calm about what he said, that Lily's dad asked him, "You're serious, aren't you?"

"Completely," said Curly. "I never joke about my business."

`"How would we earn it?" Lily asked.

Curly smiled. Then he said, "I knew we would come to this point, so we began preparing with the first clue. Do you remember what you brought me as payment?"

"The first rays of the sun in a bottle," Lily said.

"And the second payment for the next clue?"

"A picture of fire-works, including red ones," Lily added.

"Good, good," Curly said. He looked flushed as if he were very excited. "So just tell me which song refers to those two things, and you've earned it."

If Curly thought they would get it on the spot, he was disappointed. They couldn't answer. In fact, apart from a guess that the song was "Time in a Bottle" they didn't come close. Finally, Curly said, "Look. It's way too hard to do it this way. Here," he said, brandishing what looked like four tickets, "go to the ball game tonight. Relax. I get these tickets for supporting the minor league team, but I don't like going to the stadium with all its steps, and rarely use them. You had better hurry," he said, and then he stared directly into Lily's eyes. "It is bad to be late."

Lily's dad hadn't seen the look Curly had given Lily and started to say, "Well, I don't know. I hate to rush and..."

"Dad," Lily interrupted, "I really want to go. It's important." Her dad looked at her and didn't get it. He looked at Victoria's dad for support, and he just shrugged his shoulders.

"Okay, okay," he said. "Though when I wanted to go last month..." He looked at his daughter who was giving him an exasperated look, and gave up. "Okay," he said.

Chapter Five

They weren't late getting to the game – barely. They had just reached their seats and sat down when the announcer said over the loudspeakers, "Ladies and gentlemen, please stand for the national anthem."

They stood back up, and Lily's father leaned over to her before the singing began, and said, "Do you ever listen to the words? The first line could be, 'Jose, can you see?'"

The music began and Lily did in fact listen to the words. She smiled a bit at "Oh say can you see…" thinking that her father's version could be right, but she stopped smiling at the next line, "…by the dawn's early light." When the words hit "and the rocket's red glare, the bombs bursting in air," she knew she was right. She gripped her father's hand so tightly that he looked at her, a puzzled expression on her face. He said nothing until the anthem was done, and then asked her, "Now would you mind telling me why you just tried to crush my fingers?"

"'Don't you see?" Lily shouted among the noise from the crowd. "That's the song. You are the one who made me listen to the words. Well, Curly had me bring him the first rays of the sun. That is "dawn's early light!" And then the fireworks picture had to include red fireworks, remember? That's "rocket's red glare." This has got to be it. Why else would Curly want us to go to a ball game and to be sure not to be late? Because they always play the national anthem just before a ball game begins!"

It took a minute for Lily's dad to cycle her logic through his own mind, but when he had finished, he picked her up, saying, "You are right! My little Sherlock Holmes."

This had been the first game Victoria's father had ever been to and he asked to meet them later. He wanted to stay! The other three raced for their car and once there raced, well went as quickly as the law permitted, to see Curly. There was something very comforting finding him sitting by the fire, his head on his chest, when they entered.

"It must have been a quick game," he said, smiling.

"The first time I brought you "dawn's early light.""

"Yes, I guess you did," he responded.

"And the second time I brought you a picture of "the rocket's red glare," she added.

"So you did," he said.

"The song you wanted is our national anthem," she said.

"So it is," Curly responded. "But it has a name you know. It didn't become the national anthem until 1931. Before that, Francis Scott Key who wrote it couldn't very well call it the national anthem. So what did he call it?"

Lily honestly didn't know. Neither did Victoria. It was Lily's dad who said, "He named it the Star Spangled Banner, because it is a song about the flag."

Curly stood up, almost yelled out, "We have a winner!" There was a lot of celebrating and jumping around. They finally jumped themselves out, and Lily asked quietly what the piece of music was that they were going to use for the contest.

Curly responded, "Well I don't know yet. I am going to get it now. You wait here. I'll be right back." He then walked to the door to the back of the store, and giving them a wink, went through the door. Like the other time when Lily had seen him go through the door, there was an explosion of light that could be seen in the gap between the door and the floor. Then, after what only seemed like another moment, Curly came back through the door, a number of papers in his hands.

He was, as usual, smiling. And this time he was humming. It sounded to Lily that he was humming the national anthem. Her curiosity got the best of her. "Well?" she asked. "Are you going to tell us what this undiscovered piece of music is?" she asked.

"Of course, my dear," said Curly. "I have in my hands…" he said, and then paused for dramatic effect. After what seemed longer than the time he had been gone, he finally said, "Did you know that Ludwig van Beethoven had actually started sketches for a Tenth Symphony?

Lily's dad, who knew enough about classical music to know that Beethoven had only written nine symphonies, responded that he had never heard of a tenth.

"Nor would you have since he wrote it quite late and had given it to a friend with instructions that it not be made public until he had spent more time on it."

"And you somehow knew someone who knew someone who knew the friend?" Lily's father asked.

"No," said Curly, "I am the friend." His response temporarily put an end to discussion. Lily's dad looked like a fish opening and closing his mouth without speaking. Victoria managed to say, "But... but..." but no more. Of the three, only Lily believed him without any doubts.

"That's great Curly," she said, meaning it. "You know the Smythes will challenge the authenticity. What do we say when they do?"

"I was concerned with that too. I am told that his manuscripts are fairly unique. The ink strokes and so forth. But I also asked him to sign something attesting to the authenticity. He did, and here it is." With a flourish, he produced a sheet of parchment on which there were the same sort of scratched writing as on the sheets of music. He held it out and Lily took it. On the bottom was something that she could tell was a signature. Then she looked at the top of the document. It had today's date!! Lily's confidence dried up and her lip starting quivering with her effort to hold back her tears.

"But of course it is," Curly replied. "He just signed it while I was talking to him. Right after he wrote the composition that I was referring to."

"But he died a long time ago," Lily said.

"1827 to be precise," Curly said. "If you think linearly."

"I don't understand," Lily said.

"Most people think of time as being very orderly. Yesterday is always before today. Tomorrow is always after. That's wrong, Lily. If it weren't, I wouldn't have been able to travel back to 1826 to meet him."

"But Curly," Lily protested, "no one is going to believe a document dated yesterday, even if it is real. It just doesn't seem real."

"Really? Well, I accept your judgment about what people would believe. It actually was Beethoven's idea. He was intrigued by the notion of participating, as he called it, in the 21st Century."

"What about the music?" Lily asked.

"What about it?" Curly asked back.

"Is it believable or does it have some weird stuff in it as well?"

"Any respected Beethoven scholar will confirm that it is his. His stroke marks and the way he wrote music were very unique. It's just that…" Curly stopped and kicked some dust with his shoe, looking down.

"Just what?" Lily demanded.

"Well, he saw me humming. He was deaf late in life you know so he couldn't hear me. But he somehow could tell I was humming and asked me to play what I had hummed. I did. It was the Star Spangled Banner. And I could swear that the theme from our national anthem shows up in this new piece of Beethoven."

Chapter Six

Lily walked back towards where her father and Curly were standing. "Well, it is in the judge's hands now," she said. "I will tell you this much. They were impressed when I told them it was a new piece that Beethoven had been working on. If they believe it's real, it will clearly win over what the Smythes submitted."

"What did they submit?" her father asked.

"Dad, you wouldn't have heard of them. They're a rock band. Anyway, they were about to release a new album. The Smythes paid them to have the release be to the competition. Not a real contribution to humanity; unless you care that their latest album is out a week earlier than planned." Lily explained.

They returned home and waited. And waited. Finally, when they couldn't stand the waiting another minute, the phone rang. Lily answered, said, "I understand. We're on our way," and then told the rest what she had herself been told, that the competition judges wanted to announce their decision and wanted the contestants there.

When they arrived, they spotted the Smythes. At their fathers' urging, the two girls went up to the Smythes and wished them good luck. Priscilla bristled with dislike. "Fake!" she spat at them. They were spared the need for a response because at that moment they heard the young man from the competition say, "Ladies and gentlemen, may I have your attention please." Lily and Victoria made their way back to where their fathers were standing. Lily took her father's hand, and listened.

The young man continued, "Here to explain the judge's decision is Judge Driscoll, the chairman of the music department at Carnegie Mellon University, and as it turns out, a Beethoven scholar."

The judge made his way to the microphone, thanked the young man, and began. "Hello," he said, "Is this thing on?" he asked, gesturing to the microphone. Assured by the crowd that it was, he continued, "It is a rare day that one has the pleasure of discovering something new. Thanks to Lily and Victoria, this contest has given me that pleasure in the form of a manuscript of original music by the greatest composer of all times, Ludwig van Beethoven. It is most definitely genuine," he said, looking directly at the Smythes as he said this. "It has all the earmarks of Beethoven's penmanship and style. Some have questioned the modern theme that appears in this work, and in particular wonder how Beethoven knew the melody that is used as well in our national anthem. The answer is that the music used for the anthem was in fact written by an English composer named John Stafford Smith in the mid-1760's. That was some fifty years before the date of the composition by Beethoven here!" The judge went on and on, but the rest was just more reasons why the piece was genuine and so significant a discovery that weighing this against the week-early release of the rock album was "no contest." In other words, "The team of these two sweet young girls wins!"

Chapter Seven

There was a great deal of celebrating that went on. The sponsors of the contest thanked their lucky stars that the team that seemed so nice won. The girls were played up, and even had their pictures appear on cereal boxes. The publicity stopped being fun after a while. Fortunately, there was a freak accident where a motor home got washed into a river during a terrible storm, and ended up perched in the branches of a tree, and the public attention swung to this new story and away from them. By the time they went on the trip to Italy they had won, they were old news.

Lily went to see Curly just before they were to leave. She visited Curly nearly every day now, and wanted to tell him how much she would miss him, and how she would look forward to seeing him again when she came back. She entered the store and to her amazement, he was not in the chair by the fire. She couldn't see him, so she called his name. After an agonizing minute or two where she thought he had gone, she saw a flash of light under the door, and he emerged.

"Ah Lily," he said with an unusual sadness in his voice. "I was hoping you would come, for I must say goodbye."

"No!" she cried, and threw her arms around him. "I won't let you go."

"I will miss you too, my dear, but you must let me go, and I must go.'

"But why? You are my best friend," she said, meaning it.

He sighed, and pushed her gently just a few inches from him so that he could look into her eyes. "Lily, do you remember when I was telling you about travelling through time. I told you that it would be a mistake to assume that tomorrows always came after today?"

She shook her head yes, as a big tear started to roll down her cheek. He continued, "Well, think of me as coming from tomorrow. I am from what you think of as your future."

"That doesn't explain why you have to go," she said, not ready to give up.

"Lily. I came back just to meet you and to make certain you won that contest. I can't tell you about your future, other than to say you will do great things. Winning gave you a taste of how to deal with publicity. And it allowed me to confirm for some people who needed to know that you are a fine girl, the sort of person who really cares about other people."

For whatever reason, hearing him say nice things made the thought of separation even sadder. More tears rolled down her cheeks now. "Oh Lily, you are breaking my heart," he said, and tears began to form in his eyes as well. Then he said in a quiet, soothing voice, "Lily, my sweet girl, were I to stay with you, I would change your future. I wouldn't want to or mean to, but the things that you are going to learn by doing things on your own would be affected. Your future is too important to take risks that we might change it."

"Why? What is so important about my future?" she asked.

"That I can't tell you. I can only say that your future will be wonderful and mean a lot to a lot of people," he said. "Now come on, give me a kiss goodbye."

"You are going this instant?" she said, fearing the answer.

"Yes, I must. Now where is my kiss?"

She complied, he gave her a big hug, and then he walked to the door leading to the back of the store. He gave Lily a final wink, and he went through the door and was gone.

Lily ran home, and told her father that Curly had left. She told him everything, except what Curly had said about her future. She kept that part private, thinking of it only when she thought of Curly. Which happened very often.

About two days into the Italy trip, her smile returned. Thinking of Curly became a fond rather than painful memory.

The story of how she grew up has yet to be written. But Curly was right about everything else in this story. Do you think that he was wrong about Lily's future? I wouldn't bet against her.

PART V:

My father was a certifiable genius. He was a passionate artist as a youngster, and he told everyone that he was going to study art at the Cooper Union, a small private university in New York City that offered one hundred openings each for its two schools – engineering and fine arts. Admittance was by examination only. My father was taking what he thought was the art exam, and approached the proctors to ask why there was so much mathematics on the art exam. He was told that he was in fact taking the engineering exam; the art exam was the following week. He took both exams, and was admitted to both schools. Based on pressure from his mother that he would never be able to support a family from his painting, he pursued an engineering degree. The only complaint I ever heard him make about his college days was that owing to his having skipped three grades, he was only fifteen when he began college, and was therefore excluded from most of the social activities his peers engaged in. Academically, he did fine, finishing first in his class.

During World War II, he worked on airplane design. He would meet every Friday with his consultant, Charles Lindbergh, to go over the cockpit design of a navy fighter called the Vought F4U Corsair. After the war, the United States military determined to build a U.S. capability in guided missiles, and asked each of the several top weapons companies to put up two of their best people to review the captured German documents re their V-2 program. My father was one, and though he spoke not a word of German, he thought it unremarkable that he sat down and went through the German documents, solely with the aid of a German dictionary.

After the war, he became one of the top guided missile engineers in the country. He led the teams that designed and built two of the nuclear missiles in the U.S. arsenal: the Pershing missile, a highly mobile tactical nuclear missile, widely credited with deterring Russian moves against Western Europe; and the Sprint missile, an anti-ballistic missile (ABM). He was awarded the US Army's Outstanding Civilian Service Award for his work. Not bad for the son of illegal immigrants! (His mother, a Russian Jew, was denied entry at Ellis Island due to poor eyesight. She was sent back to Russia. She made the trip a second time, this time immigrating to Canada, and then slipping across the border and living the rest of her life illegally in Bridgeport, CT.)

EIGHTEENTH INTERLUDE:

A PICTURE OF MY FATHER

My father is eighty-six years old now, and his memory fails him selectively. He had never been good remembering people's names. He also has hearing problems caused by an accident during a missile test so he seldom hears the names to begin with. As a result, I was not surprised by the number of times people, mostly women of my father's age, would come up to meet "Sidney's boy," that is, me, only to have him answer my inquiry a moment later with his standard, "I have no idea what his or her name is," or the stronger variant, "I have no idea who that person is!"

There were other things he remembered too well. Being Jewish, he had a store of stories and jokes that he thought were amusing, which he shared with those he met. If you met him only once, the stories could be quite funny, even charming. Being his son, however, I had heard them so many times that I thought I could have told them myself (and plan to someday). He shared with me just recently the story of how his picture was taken by a famous photographer. It was something he had never talked about before.

The photographer's name was Philippe Halsman. My father, who couldn't remember the names of his current neighbors, professed shock that I didn't remember Halsman's name or who he was. Out came the Time Life books from the early 1960s, each volume dedicated to the most significant photographs of a particular year. In these were Halsman's wonderful portraits of Einstein, Oppenheimer, Marilyn Munroe and others. In the top drawer of his desk, I found the Halsman photograph of my father and another man, posing in front of a Pershing missile. I asked about it, and received the following history of Halsman.

Halsman had grown up in Austria, during the rise of Nazi power. When he was seventeen, his father had died tragically in a fall during a mountain climbing trip the two had taken. In pre-war Austria, this presented the opportunity to treat a situation that demanded sympathy with villainy instead. The boy was charged with murdering his father, his motive allegedly being to collect on a non-existent insurance policy that the prosecutor nonetheless described in great detail. The young Halsman was convicted and sentenced to twenty years of hard labor.

The case drew international attention, partly because of the mother's appeal to the most famous Austrian Jew of the time, Albert Einstein. Einstein used his fame to put a spotlight on the government prosecution. The government, embarrassed by the attention given to its prosecution of a young, Jewish boy using made-up facts, gave the boy a new trial. This time, the government asserted that the boy had killed his father because he had an Oedipus complex, was in love with his mother, and viewed his father as a rival. To counter this, the defense called Sigmund Freud, who testified on the boy's behalf. Once again, however, the young Halsman was convicted of murder, and was imprisoned. Finally, two years later, the outgoing president of Austria made a deal to permit the boy to escape prison, so long as he left Austria and never came back. The boy, Philippe Halsman, came to the United States, aided by Eleanor Roosevelt, and became a photographer. Years later, he took a picture of my father that I was now holding in my hands. At the time it was taken, my father was unaware of this history, discovering it several years later upon reading Einstein's autobiography.

My father was very proud of this picture, and this caused him to make an error in judgment. My father's father had left family behind in Russia when he came to this country, and my father had began corresponding with his three first cousins who lived near Kiev. He sent small gifts, and they exchanged letters and photographs, including the picture of my father taken by Halsman. The picture was spotted by the Russian secret police, which had been monitoring the mail. They descended upon the families there, and demanded that they convince my father to come to Russia for a visit. My father declined, and the families were punished: Their children were not permitted to attend Russian Universities and they were deemed ineligible for government jobs (which were most jobs in the Soviet Union at the time).

When the cold war ended, some of the Russian relatives immigrated to this country, and my father learned for the first time what sharing the Halsman photograph had done. There is irony in the fact that their two professions brought Halsman and my father together. Halsman had wanted to become an engineer but became an artist; my father had wanted to become an artist and became an engineer.

It was only because they each did so well in their second choice-careers that they met.

My father kept the Halsman photograph in his top desk drawer until he died. I found other things there as well, such as the US Army's Outstanding Civilian Service Award that we never talked about. There is a richness of life's experiences that has been lost.

My father also was far more comfortable in the world of work, where most problems had mathematical answers, to the world outside, where things got messy. It is why, when I asked him what the best day of his life had been, he said without hesitation that it was the day he found out that his team had won the Sprint contract. It is also why in his eighties, when his work finally dried up, he had nothing to replace it with.

Still, there were plenty of bright moments...

☆☆☆

NINETEENTH INTERLUDE

LEAPING LIZARDS!

As Father's Day approaches, my siblings and I search for stories that remind us of our father, who died in 2012 at the age of 92. The story of the green lizard is one of my favorites.

The prop is easy – it was one of those rubber, green lizards, 2-3 inches in length, that one might buy at the five and ten cents store. This particular one had come from our dentist as a reward for a good check-up. (It must have been won by my brother or sister.) Why the lizard became a figure of such mirth is more complicated.

It would have been a mistake to think of my father as "stern." He had a quick wit, and liked nothing better than to make people laugh. It is true that he was far more likely to employ his sense of humor in his professional life, than with his wife or three children, where he tried to be more serious.

It wasn't until years after the fact, after I had asked him to put down on paper some of his stories from work that I was able to enjoy this side of him. Like the time a colleague of his had been challenged in a room full of people for being a blowhard; i.e., for talking too much. My father had a reputation for integrity, and the colleague appealed to him for support. My father thought only a moment before issuing the perfect engineer's response: "No," he opined, "you don't talk too much, though occasionally your word to thought ratio does run a bit high."

The other thing you should know is that my father would not give his family his full attention during dinner, despite my mother's best efforts. The three children were expected to be there in the flesh, and to report on the day's experiences. My father would pretend to listen but wouldn't invest his full attention in the conversation. Rather, he would read the mail, play a word game with one of the kids, or a game of chess with me.

Perhaps it was the dissatisfaction with the level of interest my father exhibited, or perhaps it was ennui, but when the idea was floated of hiding our rubbery friend among the lettuce leaves that were piled on his plate, my mother laughed like a schoolgirl and joined the conspiracy.

One more extraneous fact you must absorb: we ate huge salads each night. I don't mean large salads. I mean that once again my mother had gotten carried away, and there was so much salad piled on each of our plates that the lizard would have ample hiding spots. After much discussion, we started the lizard's adventure a few forkfuls from the top of the salad heap, modestly hidden beneath a large leaf of Romaine.

We were all sworn to behave no differently than usual. Ha! Each of us took turns running from the room and bursting into hysterics as the fork lifted pieces of lettuce closer and closer to the lizard. My father seemed oblivious to everything, as he neared the end of the mail. Finally, without seeing it at first, he lifted the lizard from its surroundings, unaware at first that he had something very different on his fork. It was likely the different weight of the beast that caused him to notice. Finally, there was visual evidence, with my father locking into a stare with the lizard. The effect was complete, or nearly so. He became so preoccupied with getting whatever it was on his fork off, that he inadvertently seemed to give the lizard life, making it dance on the end of his fork, before it fell to the floor.

If there were ever a group of conspirators that were incapable of concealing their involvement, it was we. We hooted and hollered, we rolled on the floor laughing at the prank. Finally -- to his credit – my father figured out what had happened, and a chuckle, maybe even a full laugh, broke from his otherwise serious countenance.

☆☆☆

PART VI:

TRAVELS TO NORTH CAROLINA

I started my trips to North Carolina several years ago, at the urging of Mike Dennis, an extremely energetic pediatrician, who lived in Asheville, North Carolina. Mike was fighting Parkinson's disease, as well as the depression that affects many who have it. It is difficult, as I wrote years ago in "Silence of the Bunnies" to get through the pain and difficulties caused by the disease and realize, due to the progressive nature of the disease, that you will look back at this as the "good old days."

In any event, my writing had lifted his spirits, at least for the time, and I was doing very well with my DBS implants. He prevailed upon me to come down and speak to support groups, which I did. A few years later, we had a falling out and I lost track of him for a year or two. We re-connected, mended our fences, but I sensed something wasn't right. I heard from a mutual friend that he passed away.

This story is from happier times. I wrote it after the first trip down to North Carolina.

BLESS THEIR HEARTS

I recently traveled to Asheville, North Carolina, at the invitation of Mike Dennis, a retired pediatrician, to give talks to a number of support groups for those with Parkinson's disease. I too have PD, but I had deep brain stimulation five years ago (a remarkable procedure in which electrodes are placed in the brain) and have few visible symptoms. The idea was to give others hope by showing how well I am doing.

What I didn't count on was being so completely charmed by the circle of people surrounding Mike. He is a one-man support structure, helping those just diagnosed find their ways to get the right medical care, and giving what support he could personally.

Mike has what he calls Atypical Parkinsonism – he has severe symptoms on one side of his body, and none of the other. The result is that he must drag his non-responsive side around, using his other side to do so. Sadly, there is little or no research being done on his particular situation, so he has little hope of relief.

Despite that, he is a font of good cheer and bad jokes. He laughs harder than anyone when he tells them. His good humor is infectious, and to move among his friends is to be entertained by the constant humor and good feelings emanating from a unique group of people. There is Lucy, an effervescent lady who is a speech therapist, and Chloe, a physical therapist who ties Mike in knots in such a way that every man watching becomes jealous. There are Mary and Robert, both former singers with the Metropolitan Opera in New York, and both still active in the local community. There is Stoney, a sculptor who has been recently diagnosed with PD, and who does wondrous work with a chain saw and large lathe, bringing out the soul of wood for the rest of us to see. And there is Stoney's wife, Susan, who owns a restaurant called the Purple Onion, which serves enticing food and moderately priced wine. It also provides a haven for local talent to entertain those in attendance three nights a week.

Then there are Mason and Jennifer Thomas. Jennifer is a waitress at the Purple Onion and met Mike who frequented the place. Mike, recently divorced, was looking for someone to live-in, and give him some help doing things he is no longer able to do. Mason and Jennifer were living at the time in a cabin without running water or electricity deep in the woods. They're not hillbillies, though they would say they are. They are instead present-day replicas of Henry David Thoreau, as best I can tell. As Jennifer explains, they do not wish to be slaves to money, and therefore resist anything (including a mortgage), which would result in monthly bills. As a result, they have little but owe nothing. They work and live free from the stresses of "making ends meet." They moved in with Mike, and it seems to work for all.

Jennifer is very pretty, and makes one understand the attractiveness of spending one's life in such simple bliss. Mason is a strong personality who plays jazz guitar, paints watercolors and makes exceptional furniture. Jennifer is 36; Mason is 55. Age is not an issue, at least not now. They both want the same things and complement each other more than most couples of the same age.

I fell in love with these folk's manner of speaking. Lucy started my voyage of discovery of local idioms one afternoon by explaining that one could say virtually anything, including insults that one wouldn't think of using otherwise, so long as one attached them to the words, "Bless Her (or his) heart." For instance, one wouldn't comment on a person's propensity to perspire in gentile company, but one could, raising one's hand to one's mouth in order to shield the words from unintended recipients, say, "She sure sweats a lot for someone so skinny, bless her heart." As explained to me, the blessing relieves the speaker of all responsibility for the statement. Cool, huh?

How about, "Watch yourself on that floor; it is slicker than snot on a door knob." Or, "I'm gonna git this dinner fixed even if it hairlips every cow in Texas." The first statement is self-explanatory; the second is used to describe the certainty of the statement. Again as explained to me, "There are a whole lot of cows in Texas, and I ain't never seen one with no hairlip." Nor are these rude statements made by teenagers and looked down upon by everyone else; both of these statements are attributed by Mason to his mother. The language belongs to a group of people that are close to the earth, and have a twinkle in their eyes.

It is hard to describe the sheer delight of spending time with these gentle souls. They take an immediate interest in your life, asking about details and actually listening to the answers. And, they volunteer any information you want to hear about themselves. The result is that after a day, I felt like I knew them a week; after three and a half days, I felt like I knew them from the beginnings of time. Now I am sitting in the plane, returning to New Jersey, and my thoughts are still with my new friends. They're a lot of fun for a bunch of hillbilly hicks. Bless their hearts.

☆☆☆

More of the same…

HOW TO TALK LIKE YOU IS FROM NORTH CAROLINA

Lookit; I'ma only gonna do this if you understand that I ain't making fun of these hee-yah wonnerful folk. Got that? It's just that their manner of talking is so charming that it cries out for broader use and understanding. And that's right here's what I'm fixin to do.

A word of explanation before we begin. I said North Carolina in my title rather than South Carolina cause more people live in North Carolina, and I figured maybe I'd get lucky and more of you reading it would be from North Carolina. In truth, there ain't a rat's ass difference in how the folks talk from either state, ceptin that if you're trying to imitate someone from South Carolina it's best to slip in about twice as many grammatical mistakes as you would for someone from North Carolina.

Right. Now there's one other point that I've got to cover and then we can get started. And that is that you have got to suspend your views on what is vulgar and what isn't. Lookit, some 75-80% if all sentences spoken by folks from North Carolina have the words "Shit" or "Fuck" in them. It ain't dirty and it don't mean what you think it might mean. These are words that I call "evocative" words because they are used to capture the speaker's emotional response.

For instance, if one were to watch a runner run the hundred-yard dash, you could say, "Didja see that fella run his black ass off?" The problem, of course, is that you need a helluva lot of words to say that, and even then, you rightly can be criticized for using the phrase "black ass" even though the winner of the race clearly had one and you didn't mean nothing by it anyway. In order to avoid such misunderstandings, though, the truly modern North

Carolinian has evolved to be much more reticent, and is far more apt to comment, "Shit," upon seeing the conclusion of the race, in order to register his respect. 'Course, if the runner really did a nice job of kicking ass and taking names, the modern North Carolinian is more likely to register a stronger response, using either what I call the "Shit extender," that being to say shit but more like, "Sheeeee-i-i-it!" or the penultimate compliment, "Fuck!"

Right, so supposen you was just asked by someone whether you liked a certain girl. You could say, "Hell yeah! I mean did you see the rack on her!" Again, however, unless you are of the extremely talkative folks from around the University campuses of the state, it is far more typical to say, "Shit," (meaning anything from "no" to "yes") or "Fuck," (meaning anything from "Hell No!" to "Hell Yes!"). The exact meaning of the words must be derived from, anybody? That's right, the context. For instance, if the speaker says "shit" or "fuck" in a negative manner, then it's no; if in a positive manner, then it's yes.

Okay, let's take you out for some practice. Fortunately, there are a group of friends meeting for a cider party about three miles out of town. We come a bit late, and greet the hosts who aren't really a couple. She adores him, but you happen to know that he hit on your babe when you were recovering from that auto accident last summer.

The sonofabitch speaks first, "Well lookee what the cat dragged in. Howdee Laverne. Howdee, Butch." He knows your name ain't Butch and he knows that you don't like being called Butch. He is trying to put you down.

"Shit," you say in response [meaning here that you know exactly what he is up to.]

"C'mon in, and try some of Skeeter's cider." He calls his girlfriend Skeeter for some reason. He pours us each a cup and we take sips. It's very good.

"Fuck, that's really good," Laverne blurts out [meaning "thank you. It tastes quite good."]

"Fuckin A," our host (the sonofabitch) responds meaning, "Thank you," with a hint of, "Hey, want to dump your loser boyfriend and get laid?"

Anyhow, you decide to tell a story to change the subject. For some reason, it is accepted in the Carolinas that the better stories all have to be out of context, meaning they have nothing to do with the conversation that precedes the story. "Ya know," you say, "that reminds me of a story I heard, about some professor who takes a young girl and completely changes the girl's life by changing the way she talks."

"Shit," the sonofabitch responded sarcastically, "that's about the dumbest story I ever hear-ed. Why, how you talk ain't important. If it was, well, y'know I don't talk real purty. How the hell would I hold down just about the most important job in these parts in law enforcement?" The man was a part time, substitute private cop who worked at Woolworth's Tuesday and Thursday evenings, and was being considered for an even bigger job at Target.

"Yessirreee Bob," his girlfriend adds, "and Mister, I done heard that story of your'n before, though the professor didn't teach her no language; he invented flubber, a mysterious substance that made white boys able to jump nearly as high as colored boys!"

She cackled what was undoubtedly a laugh, before being grabbed from behind by a now-effusive sonofabitch, who winked at me while cupping her breasts in his massive hands. "Shit fella, you woulda had me with that story only I got me the most smart gal that a man would want and she nailed you!"

I thought about trying to tell him that she was mixed up and there were really two movies, both including professors, and that in one of them, the professor did teach a young woman to speak better. Ignorance, though, is a small price to pay for the joy these two were feeling. I swallowed the longer thought, said an admiring, "shit!", and got the fuck out of Dodge. My one consolation was to hum softly the song, "The Rain in Spain" as I walked out the door.

☆☆☆

Once I decided to move, it was a simple matter of selling my existing house, figure out where I want to live, build or buy a home, decide what possessions I wanted to keep, move those possessions to the place I chose, etc. etc. etc. Fortunately, you meet some interesting people along the way. Billy, as you can tell, was one of my favorites.

TWENTY-SECOND INTERLUDE:

BILLY AND THE REYNOLDS MANSION

Billy is a historian, curator, and innkeeper. Not to mention gardener, beekeeper, and day (and night) laborer. He has become a master of so many trades because he has had to in order to do what he has done --- preserve for the rest of us a piece of American history: the Reynolds Mansion in Asheville, North Carolina.

My finding the Mansion was a piece of pure serendipity. For a variety of reasons, I was looking for a new place to live. I reside currently in New Jersey, which is a very expensive a place to live. I pay more than $12,000 in real estate taxes on my three-bedroom condo, about $10,000 more than I would pay for a comparable residence in a place like Asheville. Now that my daughter is college bound it was time for me to look for a home outside New Jersey.

My brother had recently relocated to Asheville, and I decided to visit him to see whether it was the sort of place in which I would like to "retire." His place was still filled with unpacked boxes from his move, and he recommended I stay elsewhere during my visit. The Reynolds Mansion, a bed and breakfast not more than a stone's throw from where he was staying, was the obvious choice.

In other words, I stumbled onto this jewel of a place without a shred of research or intent. I had no inkling that I was about to meet "Billy," the magician who breathes life into the place and makes it what it is.

The building itself, a large square structure made of red brick, is but the tip of the iceberg. It was built by slaves in 1847, one of only seven brick houses built before the civil war that still exists! It survived by the narrowest of margins, falling into such a state of disrepair that plans were to knock it down, despite its designation as a historical building. The only thing that saved it was that Billy, a former executive at United Healthcare, stepped forward and bought the place, committing to use his own funds to restore it. He had had a lifetime dream of running a bed and breakfast, and saw in the ramshackle remains the potential of something great.

The historical designation is both a blessing and a curse. State law mandates that those places so designated be rehabilitated in strict accordance with the original, raising added challenges to anyone who wants to rehabilitate such a place. That means, for example, that since the original building did not have handrails on the stairs leading up to the house, they could not be installed now.

Restoring the mansion was no simple task. The building had been abandoned some seven years earlier, and everything had fallen into disrepair. Ivy was growing on the interior walls in several rooms, the enormous porch around the house had rotted and collapsed, part of the roof had collapsed and the entire inside of the house was covered by black soot, because of the coal that had been used in the fireplaces.

Billy attacked the place with a passion born of love, insight into the possible and sheer lunacy. Three crews worked collectively twenty-four hours a day, seven days a week for eighteen months doing the restoration. Working under the guidance of state-appointed restoration experts, the building was restored faithfully as much as possible. Lumber to rebuild the porch was hand-milled, because modern mills no longer made lumber with the required dimensions. Paintings were lovingly restored by an expert in Washington, D.C., who cleaned the black soot from their surfaces and made other repairs. Still other details could not be perfectly replicated. An example of this was the stairs. A slave named Amos had built the original stairways in the house. Though uneducated, he had skills that can no longer be found in modern workers, and the restored stairs are not quite up to the same standards as were the original.

At the same time that the structure was being restored, Billy also began contacting members of the Reynolds family in a quest to reacquire the original furnishings that had been removed from the house over the many generations that the family had lived there. Daniel Reynolds, brother of R.J. Reynolds, the tobacco tycoon, had built the house. After Daniel, another four generations of family members owned the house. This included Mamie Reynolds, a woman of fantastic wealth who at one time owned the Hope Diamond, the Star of the East Diamond and the Star of India Diamond, and, Adeline Reynolds, a woman of modest means who sold off everything not nailed down, including the dining table and all but five of the fifteen hundred acres the house had originally had.

Because the various members of the Reynolds family were so generous, returning all sorts of items, staying at the Mansion is like staying at a museum. Behind every item is a story, and Billy knows them all.

By far the best time of the day when staying there is the hour or so from 9 – 10 a.m. That is the time for breakfast. Not only is the food sensational, made from the freshest of ingredients (eggs come from Billy's chickens; fruits and vegetables primarily from his organic garden), but this also is the time when Billy joins his guests and tells them stories about the place. My favorite stories are the ones about the ghosts that have been sighted at various times, but all are entertaining. You want more? Then visit yourself!

I have been spoiled. This was more than a place to stay; my stay at the Mansion was the highlight of my trip. I could no more think of staying somewhere else when visiting Asheville than I could fly there with my own wings. The Reynolds Mansion is a gem, made that way by its master jeweler, Billy and his wonderful staff. You owe it to yourself to stay there.

PART VII:

Talking about politics seems to stimulate more wars than under-standing. It is why I try avoiding too much familiarity with the news. If I had more knowledge of what was going on in the world, people would expect me to have an opinion about things, and therein lies danger. Still, despite my determination to avoid getting sucked in, there are times when the provocation becomes so intense that some sort of reaction against "it" becomes unavoidable. Like when the Texas School Board directed that Thomas Jefferson be de-emphasized in favor of John Calvin.

TWENTY-THIRD INTERLUDE:

THE TEXAS TALIBAN

George Washington crossed the Rio Grande, ambushing the French at Bastogne. Right? Unburdened by the liberal rant of the Supreme Court, he also conducted a prayer beforehand for his troops, in which he invoked Jesus' name to aid his cause.

Hopefully, you've identified the numerous errors in the above. Washington crossed the Delaware River to attack the Hessians, German mercenaries fighting for the British, at Trenton, New Jersey. Bastogne was a key city in the World War II Battle of the Bulge, where American troops withstood a German counter-offen-sive. As for the prayer, Washington was a deist who never in his writings referred to Jesus Christ. It is unlikely that he would have done so here.

Many teenagers can't identify the various mistakes in the paragraph. It's not that they're stupid; the problem is that they are taught only a superficial gloss of American history.

Correcting this is complicated by an active and growing anti-democratic movement that seems bent on interfering with a fact-based education. For example, the Texas school board earlier this year required that references to Thomas Jefferson should be removed from textbooks used in that state and replaced with references to John Calvin.

Calvin was a sixteenth century French cleric. He had a low opinion of women ("Yet consider now, whether women are not quite past sense or reason, when they want to rule over men."), and of Jews ("Their rotten and unbending stiffneckedness deserves that they be oppressed unendingly...and that they die in their misery without the sympathy of anyone."). He also used his authority to murder a number of people, including opponents or women he accused of witchcraft.

Jefferson was a central figure in the American Revolution, and the author of the Declaration of Independence. In words as elegant as any that have been written in the political arena, Jefferson wrote:

> *"We hold these truths to be self-evident, that all men are created equal, that they are endowed by their creator with certain unalienable rights, that among these are life, liberty, and the pursuit of happiness, -- that to secure these rights governments are instituted among men, deriving their just powers from the consent of the governed — that whenever any form*

of government become destructive of these ends, it is the right of the people to alter or abolish it, and to institute new government, laying its foundation on such principles...[that] shall seem most likely to effect their safety and happiness."

So why did the Texas school board replace Jefferson with Calvin? Well, I have not mentioned a grievous sin Jefferson committed: he like virtually all of our founding fathers believed in the separation of church and state. In fact, Jefferson coined the phrase. Our founding fathers remembered the religious persecution in Europe, and wanted this country to be different. For that reason, the First Amendment of the Constitution reads in part:

"Congress shall pass no law respecting the establishment of religion, or prohibiting the free exercise thereof..."

The Texas school board members who supported the removal of Jefferson reject the notion that this country is and has always been secular. They are like another group that also embraces the notion of state-sponsored religion – the Taliban. The Taliban horrify us because they believe in government-imposed religion, and are prepared to kill those who disagree. True, the school board does not use the same tactics, but make no mistake, these "Texas Taliban" are dangerous because they blend ignorance, intolerance, and political power.

The best way to combat them is education, for when their nonsense is held up to the truth, they end up looking silly. That means not tolerating politically motivated censorship of textbooks. If we lose our grounding in truth, their claims about Washington crossing whatever river they want him to cross become more believable, as do their claims that Constitutional text doesn't exist when it clearly does.

By the way, you are aware, aren't you, that among Abraham Lincoln's accomplishments was the establishment of the zip code system, something he did near the end of the Civil War to assist the pony express. In fact, the very first piece of mail using a zip code was delivered to him at his summer house in Gettysburg, Pennsylvania, at his "Gettysburg address..." (Shhh, I think I have the school board leaning...).

☆ ☆ ☆

Or upon the occasion of actually listening to some vacuous lyrics on the radio...

Twenty-Fourth Interlude:

The Day the Music Became Self-Absorbed

I am like every middle-aged parent, wondering why the music of today just isn't as good as the music of my day. And like every middle-aged parent, I want to say, "No really, I know my parents thought the same thing and they were wrong! But I am right!"

Let me first establish a baseline: I was born in 1952, and thus was a teenager during the 1960s. If there ever were a golden age of popular music, that was it. We had the Beatles, the Stones, the Grateful Dead, Simon & Garfunkel, and Bob Dylan, to name only a few. The music celebrated fun – songs like "I Want to Hold Your Hand" didn't get too deep into the human condition. But musicians also were willing to take risks with lyrics, questioning the establishment and fomenting rebellion against war, inequality, and just about any other issue of the day.

Lyrics were important, and in many cases were poetry set to song. Not every song had a meaning, but enough did so that the music helped those unhappy with what was going on in the world galvanize their feelings into protest. Woodstock happened. Is it any wonder?

Look at Dylan's lyrics from Blowing in the Wind:

"How many times must a man look up

Before he can see the sky?

Yes, 'n how many ears must one man have

Before he can hear people cry?

Yes, 'n how many deaths will it take till he knows

That too many people have died?

The answer, my friend, is blowin' in the wind

The answer is blowin' in the wind."

Music was a political force. And it helped change this nation, for the better. It is a medium that reaches young people like no other; when the musicians they admire attack social injustice, it makes an impact! Who today in the music world is willing to pick up Dylan's legacy and write songs that make a difference?

Today, musicians seem to care about getting rich and getting laid. I gave my 13-year old daughter the assignment of collecting the lyrics from about a half dozen popular hits. I don't mean to pick on the artists that she selected – there is nothing wrong with either getting rich or getting laid, and I enjoy the songs that I mention below. My point only is that this is not meaningful stuff in any social or political sense.

Take Taio Cruz' lyrics to Dynamite:

"I came to dance, dance, dance

"I hit the floor

'Cause that's my plans, plans, plans, plans

I'm wearing all my favorite brands

Give me space for my hands, hands, hands, hands

You, you

Cause it goes on and on

And it goes on and on and on.

I throw my hands up in the air sometimes

Saying AYO

Gotta Let Go

I wanna celebrate and live my life

Saying AYO

Baby, let's go."

Or how about OMG by Usher:

"I fell in love when I seen her on the dance floor

She was dancing sexy, pop, pop, popping, Dropping,

droping low

Never ever has a lady hit me on the first sight

This was something special, this was just like Dynamite.

Honey got a booty like pow, pow, pow

Honey got some boobies like wow, oh wow."

And so on. The point I am making, albeit unscientifically, is that today's lyrics celebrate hedonism. That's not bad; but it's not all there is. Where is the power of music used to stop wars, or fight social injustice?

Where, for the love of God, is John Lennon:

"Imagine no possessions

I wonder if you can

No need for greed or hunger

A brotherhood of man

Imagine all the people

Sharing all the world

You may say I'm a dreamer

But I'm not the only one

I hope some day you'll join us

And the world will live as one."

Look around you. It's not as if we have run out of issues that tear at one's soul. What has happened to music? What has happened to us?

☆ ☆ ☆

Or perhaps when people start arguing about the causes of the health care crisis without coming close to the real reasons...

Graham Crackers and the Secret to Lower Medical Costs

I am a showcase for the marvels of modern medicine: I have two electrodes in my brain wired to two controllers in my chest to control the symptoms of Parkinson's disease. I have another three pieces of metal - a ring, a stent, and a defibrillator -- in my chest, implanted in three different operations in order to keep my heart going. I've also had less major surgeries on my hand, my knee, and two on my right foot. The combined cost for all of these procedures was around a million dollars.

It is the conventional wisdom among conservatives that health care cost increases are caused by government regulation or attorneys who sue doctors, making malpractice premiums go up. It is the equivalent wisdom of liberals that it is the fault of rapacious insurance companies. No doubt there are examples of both, but in my experience, which is considerable, the fault lies far more with the service providers – including doctors and hospitals.

During my brain surgery at Robert Wood Johnson hospital, the surgeon had three young doctors observe to gain experience. One of them was asked to help perform calculations, involving adding numbers together, to determine the proper drilling coordinates. The young man someday might prove to be a good doctor, but he couldn't add. My insurance company was billed three thousand dollars a piece for the attendance of these "surgical assistants." Uh-huh.

I am a mess. I have Parkinson's disease, heart problems, and occasionally I suffer injuries I can't blame on genetics - like cutting my hand on a broken ceramic bowl I was getting for late-night ice cream. The cut became infected and I had hand surgery, following which I was hospitalized for three days. The hospital didn't stock my Parkinson's drugs so I used my own, which I take four times a day. The helpful nurses took the jar from me, and four times a day, gave me back a pill. The hospital charge for this "coordination of medication" was $50 a day, a small charge lost in the total bill, but larceny all the same.

Following a heart attack on July 4, 2009, I was hospitalized about two weeks. The hospital used all the latest technology, including inducing a coma and lowering my body temperature to preserve the health of my organs. Whatever they did, it worked and I am eternally grateful. The cost of the stay lies in a mysterious maze of bills, but was somewhere between $300,000 and $400,000, all in. Of this, most was legitimate, or at least I think so. But some clearly was not. There were at least a half dozen specialists, doctors whom I never remember seeing, who charged a consultation charge of several hundred dollars a day for each day I was in the hospital. Not a few days; but every day. I suspect most of these charges resulted from brief "fly-bys," brief visits of no more than five minutes where the specialist either looked at my chart on days when he was at the hospital for other reasons, or called, and asked a question or two when he wasn't. Sure, some of the doctors were helpful some of the time, but there was clearly excess billing here.

When one does come out of a coma, there are a number of issues to deal with. One of them is that you have been fed intravenously for so long a patient may have difficulty swallowing. The protocol used by Morristown Memorial hospital to determine a patient's ability to swallow is to require the patient to drink barium, and then use x-rays to watch the progress of the slime as it is swallowed. The hospital claims this is completely safe, though the literature does point out that some patients suffer severe constipation.

I refused to take the barium based on my belief that one is better off not drinking heavy metal without good reason. The hospital refused to give me real food until I did. Finally, a wonderful doctor broke the impasse with a graham cracker. She brought it to me, told me to eat it, and watched as I did so. She then opined that I could swallow, and I was allowed to eat real food again.

I don't know how much the hospital charges for the barium test, though the literature says that the cost of the procedure ranges from $90 to 120, excluding the costs of the people, of which there were six or seven involved, or the depreciation of the various monitors used to track the slime as it passed the way down the hatch. Using the usual hospital multiplier, the procedure is likely to run several thousand dollars. In contrast, the "graham cracker test" costs about ten cents, doesn't require the use of any special x-ray equipment, and doesn't present any intestinal issues. Why then is the standard routine to require the barium drink?

Following my release from the hospital, I had to wear a "defibrilla-tor vest" for six days prior to having the device installed in my chest. The rent for the vest for one week was three thousand dollars! The cost to make the vest has got to be less than that, but who has the time or the ability to shop around?

The problem is that my experience is not unique or even exceptional. We've become conditioned to the outrageous billing and don't make a fuss because we don't have to pay – insurance companies do. Then, when employers and insurance companies can no longer cover the spiraling costs and have cut back their coverage, we react predict-ably – we got angry with the insurance companies. There is so much wrong with the health care system that even were all providers to become suddenly honest, it would not fix the problem. But it is a start and would help. I suggest that those who provide the services that trigger the bills for health care should take a look in the mirror, and while doing so ask themselves the question: assume for a moment that this is a bill to your mother who would want you to sit down and explain each item contributing to the total bill. Would the bill be the same as it is now?

☆☆☆

EPILOGUE:

My father brought his own life to an end, by directing that his food and medicine be withheld. He was not in pain; he was bored. He had chosen to live on the West Coast, despite the fact that all three of his grandkids lived on the East Coast. He was not a happy man.

His work, which had been the center of his life, had gradually dried up. He had worked as a consultant beginning at age 65 when he retired, and did this for a number of years. But over time, his inability to hear well made it difficult for others to work with him, and the work disappeared. Without his work, he was without his love and ended up lonely and without something to make it all worthwhile.

To some extent, his loneliness was a function of his longevity – he lived to a ripe old age of 92, which is another way of saying that most of the people who knew him were long since dead.

How do I avoid going down this same path? Clearly, I have demonstrated that the issue of longevity will not be something I need to worry about. But assume for the sake of argument that I live past the time where I still get enjoyment from writing down my thoughts and assume further that I lose the five or ten people most responsible for keeping me connected to the human race. Then what? I have been doing this all wrong! I have been allowing my health issues, which are considerable, to keep me on the sidelines. Why? It seems a dumb idea. Surely, there must be women – my nature compels this limitation – that would choose me over the loneliness they are experiencing.

As I write this, I realize that I also fear that by revealing my need for others I invite people who I don't really love to enter the game, and declare that they have solved my problem! The fact is that what I really want is an imbalance – a situation where I can attract women who are healthier and more attractive than I. Most people who are not healthier than I are already dead! It's really a very simple problem: to avoid a situation where I continue living without friendship, I need to find attractive women who desire or at least don't mind, drooling Parkinsonian men with weak hearts and little or no muscular coordination. It's a piece of friggin' cake!

So long as I do this with honesty, is there really a reason not to get in there and mix it up? (At least until 8:30 p.m., when my energy starts running low?)

Good Grief! I think I'd better think it out again!

Dan Stark

May 24, 2020